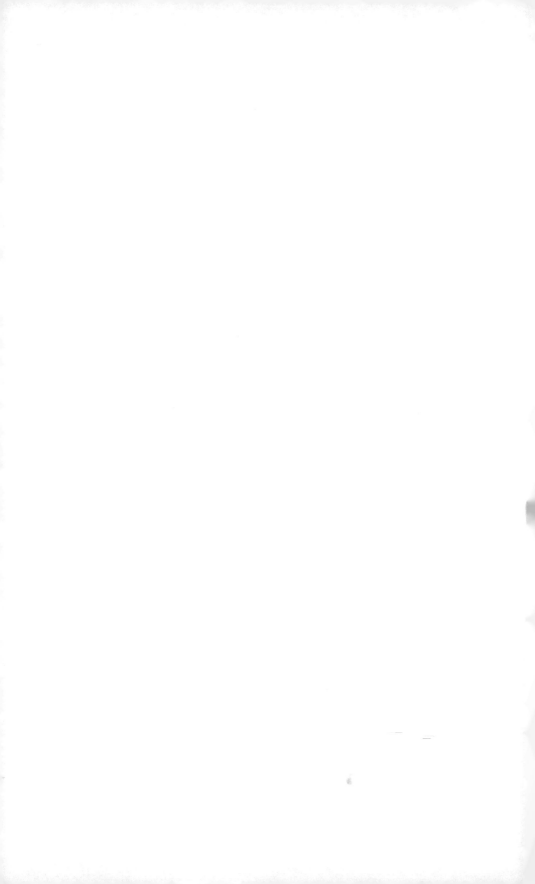

Stochastic Dynamics for Systems Biology

CHAPMAN & HALL/CRC
Mathematical and Computational Biology Series

Aims and scope:

This series aims to capture new developments and summarize what is known over the entire spectrum of mathematical and computational biology and medicine. It seeks to encourage the integration of mathematical, statistical, and computational methods into biology by publishing a broad range of textbooks, reference works, and handbooks. The titles included in the series are meant to appeal to students, researchers, and professionals in the mathematical, statistical and computational sciences, fundamental biology and bioengineering, as well as interdisciplinary researchers involved in the field. The inclusion of concrete examples and applications, and programming techniques and examples, is highly encouraged.

Series Editors

N. F. Britton
Department of Mathematical Sciences
University of Bath

Xihong Lin
Department of Biostatistics
Harvard University

Hershel M. Safer
School of Computer Science
Tel Aviv University

Maria Victoria Schneider
European Bioinformatics Institute

Mona Singh
Department of Computer Science
Princeton University

Anna Tramontano
Department of Physics
University of Rome La Sapienza

Proposals for the series should be submitted to one of the series editors above or directly to:
CRC Press, Taylor & Francis Group
3 Park Square, Milton Park
Abingdon, Oxfordshire OX14 4RN
UK

Published Titles

Algorithms in Bioinformatics: A Practical Introduction
Wing-Kin Sung

Bioinformatics: A Practical Approach
Shui Qing Ye

Biological Computation
Ehud Lamm and Ron Unger

Biological Sequence Analysis Using the SeqAn C++ Library
Andreas Gogol-Döring and Knut Reinert

Cancer Modelling and Simulation
Luigi Preziosi

Cancer Systems Biology
Edwin Wang

Cell Mechanics: From Single Scale-Based Models to Multiscale Modeling
Arnaud Chauvière, Luigi Preziosi, and Claude Verdier

Clustering in Bioinformatics and Drug Discovery
John D. MacCuish and Norah E. MacCuish

Combinatorial Pattern Matching Algorithms in Computational Biology Using Perl and R
Gabriel Valiente

Computational Biology: A Statistical Mechanics Perspective
Ralf Blossey

Computational Hydrodynamics of Capsules and Biological Cells
C. Pozrikidis

Computational Neuroscience: A Comprehensive Approach
Jianfeng Feng

Computational Systems Biology of Cancer
Emmanuel Barillot, Laurence Calzone, Philippe Hupé, Jean-Philippe Vert, and Andrei Zinovyev

Data Analysis Tools for DNA Microarrays
Sorin Draghici

Differential Equations and Mathematical Biology, Second Edition
D.S. Jones, M.J. Plank, and B.D. Sleeman

Dynamics of Biological Systems
Michael Small

Engineering Genetic Circuits
Chris J. Myers

Exactly Solvable Models of Biological Invasion
Sergei V. Petrovskii and Bai-Lian Li

Game-Theoretical Models in Biology
Mark Broom and Jan Rychtář

Gene Expression Studies Using Affymetrix Microarrays
Hinrich Göhlmann and Willem Talloen

Genome Annotation
Jung Soh, Paul M.K. Gordon, and Christoph W. Sensen

Glycome Informatics: Methods and Applications
Kiyoko F. Aoki-Kinoshita

Handbook of Hidden Markov Models in Bioinformatics
Martin Gollery

Introduction to Bioinformatics
Anna Tramontano

Introduction to Bio-Ontologies
Peter N. Robinson and Sebastian Bauer

Introduction to Computational Proteomics
Golan Yona

Introduction to Proteins: Structure, Function, and Motion
Amit Kessel and Nir Ben-Tal

An Introduction to Systems Biology: Design Principles of Biological Circuits
Uri Alon

Kinetic Modelling in Systems Biology
Oleg Demin and Igor Goryanin

Knowledge Discovery in Proteomics
Igor Jurisica and Dennis Wigle

Published Titles (continued)

Managing Your Biological Data with Python
Allegra Via, Kristian Rother, and Anna Tramontano

Meta-analysis and Combining Information in Genetics and Genomics
Rudy Guerra and Darlene R. Goldstein

Methods in Medical Informatics: Fundamentals of Healthcare Programming in Perl, Python, and Ruby
Jules J. Berman

Modeling and Simulation of Capsules and Biological Cells
C. Pozrikidis

Niche Modeling: Predictions from Statistical Distributions
David Stockwell

Normal Mode Analysis: Theory and Applications to Biological and Chemical Systems
Qiang Cui and Ivet Bahar

Optimal Control Applied to Biological Models
Suzanne Lenhart and John T. Workman

Pattern Discovery in Bioinformatics: Theory & Algorithms
Laxmi Parida

Python for Bioinformatics
Sebastian Bassi

Quantitative Biology: From Molecular to Cellular Systems
Sebastian Bassi

Spatial Ecology
Stephen Cantrell, Chris Cosner, and Shigui Ruan

Spatiotemporal Patterns in Ecology and Epidemiology: Theory, Models, and Simulation
Horst Malchow, Sergei V. Petrovskii, and Ezio Venturino

Statistical Methods for QTL Mapping
Zehua Chen

Statistics and Data Analysis for Microarrays Using R and Bioconductor, Second Edition
Sorin Drăghici

Stochastic Dynamics for Systems Biology
Christian Mazza and Michel Benaïm

Stochastic Modelling for Systems Biology, Second Edition
Darren J. Wilkinson

Structural Bioinformatics: An Algorithmic Approach
Forbes J. Burkowski

The Ten Most Wanted Solutions in Protein Bioinformatics
Anna Tramontano

Chapman & Hall/CRC Mathematical and Computational Biology Series

Stochastic Dynamics for Systems Biology

Christian Mazza

University of Fribourg
Switzerland

Michel Benaïm

University of Neuchâtel
Switzerland

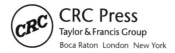

CRC Press
Taylor & Francis Group
Boca Raton London New York

CRC Press is an imprint of the
Taylor & Francis Group, an **informa** business

A CHAPMAN & HALL BOOK

Cover Image: Marie Vieli, "untitled" acrylic on paper 24 x 30 cm.

CRC Press
Taylor & Francis Group
6000 Broken Sound Parkway NW, Suite 300
Boca Raton, FL 33487-2742

© 2014 by Taylor & Francis Group, LLC
CRC Press is an imprint of Taylor & Francis Group, an Informa business

No claim to original U.S. Government works

ISBN 13: 978-1-4665-1493-5 (hbk)

Visit the Taylor & Francis Web site at
http://www.taylorandfrancis.com

and the CRC Press Web site at
http://www.crcpress.com

Contents

Preface   xi

I   Dynamics of reaction networks: Markov processes   1

1   Reaction networks: introduction   **3**

1.1   Introduction to modelling: a self-regulated gene   4

1.2   Birth and death processes to model basic chemical reactions   9

    1.2.1   Degradation   9

    1.2.2   A basic transcriptional unit   11

    1.2.3   Conversion   17

1.3   Some results on the self-regulated gene   20

    1.3.1   The case of constant g and κ   22

2   Continuous-time Markov chains   **27**

2.1   Introduction   27

    2.1.1   Birth and death processes   28

    2.1.2   The Kolmogorov equation associated with birth and death processes   28

    2.1.3   The Poisson process   31

2.2   General time-continuous Markov chains   32

    2.2.1   Spectral properties*   35

    2.2.2   Jump chain and holding times   38

    2.2.3   Convergence to equilibrium   40

2.3   Some important Markov chains   43

    2.3.1   The Metropolis-Hastings chain   43

    2.3.2   A Metropolis chain on the d-cube*   45

2.4   Two-time-scale stochastic simulations*   46

II   Illustrations from systems biology   51

3   First-order chemical reaction networks   **53**

3.1   Reaction networks   53

3.2   Linear first-order reaction networks   54

3.3   Statistical descriptors for linear rate functions   57

3.4   Open and closed conversion systems   59

3.5   Illustration: Intrinsic noise in gene regulatory networks   . . .   60

4   Biochemical pathways   **65**

4.1   Stochastic fluctuations in metabolic pathways   65

4.2   Signalling networks   69

5   Binding processes and transcription rates   **77**

5.1   Positive and negative control   78

5.2   Binding probabilities   79

5.3   Gibbs-Boltzmann distributions   83

5.4   Site-specific Hill coefficients   85

5.5   Cooperativity in the microstate*   86

5.6   The sigmoidal nature of the binding curve*   87

5.7   Cooperativity in the Hill sense   89

5.8 $\eta_H(v)$ as an indicator of cooperativity   92

5.9   The cooperativity index   93

5.10 Macroscopic cooperativity   95

5.11 The case $N = 3$*   96

5.12 Transcription rates for basic models   99

5.13 A genetic switch: regulation by λ phage repressor 102

6   Kinetics of binding processes   **109**

6.1   A mathematical model of eukaryotic gene activation 110

6.2   Steady state distribution of more general binding processes . 117

7   Transcription factor binding at nucleosomal DNA   **119**

7.1   Competition between nucleosomes and TF 119

7.2   Nucleosome-mediated cooperativity between TF 120

8   Signalling switches   **131**

8.1   Ordered phosphorylation 132

8.2   Unordered phosphorylation 133

III   A short course on dynamical systems   **137**

9   Differential equations, flows and vector fields   **139**

9.1   Some examples 139

      9.1.1   Malthus and Verhulst equations 139

      9.1.2   Predators-Preys systems: The Lotka-Volterra model . 140

9.2 Vector fields and differential equations 142
9.3 Existence and uniqueness theorems 142
    9.3.1 A global existence criterion 144
9.4 Higher order and nonautonomous equations 145
9.5 Flow and phase portrait 146
    9.5.1 Phase portrait 148
    9.5.2 The variational equation 150
        9.5.2.1 Liouville formula 150

10 Equilibria, periodic orbits and limit cycles   **153**
10.1 Equilibria, periodic orbits and invariant sets 153
10.2 Alpha and omega limit sets 154
    10.2.1 Limit cycles 155
    10.2.2 Heteroclinic cycle: The May and Leonard example . . 155
10.3 The Poincaré-Bendixson theorem 159
10.4 Chaos 159
    10.4.1 Lotka-Volterra and chaos 161
10.5 Lyapunov functions 162
10.6 Attractors 163
10.7 Stability in autonomous systems 164
10.8 Application to Lotka-Volterra equations 165
    10.8.1 Lotka-Volterra with limited growth 165
    10.8.2 Lotka-Volterra in dimension n 166

11 Linearisation   **169**
11.1 Linear differential equations 169
    11.1.1 Hyperbolic matrices, sources, sinks and saddles 171
    11.1.2 Two dimensional linear systems 173
11.2 Linearization and stable manifolds 176
    11.2.1 Nonlinear sinks 177
    11.2.2 The stable manifold theorem 178
    11.2.3 The Hartmann-Grobman linearization theorem* . . . 181
    11.2.4 The May and Leonard model (the end) 181

IV   Linear noise approximation   **183**

12 Density dependent population processes and the linear noise approximation   **185**
12.1 A law of large numbers 185
12.2 Illustration: bistable behaviour of self-regulated genes 190
12.3 Epigenetics and multistationarity 191

12.4 Gaussian approximation   193
    12.4.1 Steady state approximations   197
12.5 Illustration: attenuation of noise using negative feedback loops
    in prokaryotic transcription   199

13 Mass action kinetics   **205**
13.1 Deterministic mass action kinetics and the deficiency zero
    theorem*   207
13.2 Stochastic mass action kinetics   212
13.3 Extension to more general dynamics   216

V   Appendix   **219**

A Self-regulated genes   **221**
A.1 Dimerisation   221
    A.1.1 The invariant measure   221
    A.1.2 Computing the moments of the invariant measure . .   222
A.2 Transcription with fast dimerisation   223
    A.2.1 Inclusion of negative feedback   226
A.3 Steady state distribution: the method of transfer matrices . .   226
    A.3.1 Stochastic simulations with MATLAB®   230

**B Asymptotic behaviour of the solutions to time-continuous
Lyapunov equations**   **237**
B.1 Time-continuous Lyapunov equations   237
B.2 Asymptotically autonomous dynamical systems   238

Bibliography   **243**

Index   **257**

Preface

This book introduces time-continuous Markov chain modelling generic stochastic dynamics from systems biology, and shows how Markov chain models of biochemical reaction networks can provide insight into biological processes. This work should be useful for researchers in computational biology and bioinformatics, also for applied mathematicians and scientists willing to enter into the emerging field of systems biology. Most of the mathematical models use tools from Markov chain theory. Our approach considers a smooth way of treating these notions, using examples and illustrations from systems biology. We put in boxes either the assumed to be known mathematical notions, or some facts from advanced mathematics, the latter being explained in the main text in simple terms. More mathematically advanced sections are highlighted by stars. We have also included new material which should help make links between various notions of interest for binding processes.

Chapter 1 focuses on stochastic models of basic chemical reactions which are used to model the dynamics of self-regulated genes. These basic regulatory modules are the building blocks of many gene networks, and can exhibit bistable behaviours. Chapter 2 provides notions from time-continuous Markov chain theory, which are relevant to the rest of the book. Part II illustrates the use of time-continuous Markov chains for modelling phenomena of interest in systems biology. Chapter 3 introduces first-order linear chemical reaction networks, which are often used as first modelling frameworks. They permit us to get ideas on the behaviour of gene network intrinsic noise. Chapter 4 is a brief introduction to metabolic and signalling pathways. One shows how models from probability theory and statistical mechanics lead to a better comprehension of such pathways, which are instrumental for the cellular signal processing system.

Transcription networks are approached in chapter 5. The first part of this chapter focuses on binding processes where regulatory proteins or transcription factors bind to regulatory regions like promoters to enhance or prevent gene expression. The literature often considers models of transcription rates like Hill functions; we show how notions from statistical mechanics permit us to explain such choices. A central part of this chapter deals with the notion of cooperativity, where the binding of a molecule at some site influences the binding of molecules at other sites. Classical moment inequalities are used to shed light on the cooperative behaviours, by explaining why binding curves often have an S-shape. Chapter 6 proposes chemical kinetics for thermodynamical models of current use in biophysics, and provides a precise modelling approach to eukaryotic gene activation. Chapter 7 focuses on the indirect cooperative effects which emerge as a consequence of the competition for binding between transcription factors and nucleosomes. Chapter 8 shows how phosphorylation processes can lead to strong signalling switches.

Part III provides a short course on dynamical systems for scientists having basic knowledge of differential calculus. We have included this material since many models from systems biology use ordinary differential equations (o.d.e.) as a basic modelling framework. Some of this material is used in part IV, chapter 12, which deals with the so-called linear noise approximation. This modelling tool approximates complex nonlinear stochastic dynamics by gaussian processes, which are drifted by o.d.e. We give the precise mathematical results without proofs, and illustrate the use of such methods for studying propagation of noise in gene networks. Chapter 13 provides classic and more recent results on mass action kinetics, and shows how the associated time-continuous Markov chains are strongly related to their deterministic counterparts.

The authors warmly thank Louis-Félix Bersier, Andreas Conzelmann, Jean-Pierre Gabriel, Georges Klein, Yvan Velenik and Claudio di Virgilio for careful reading of parts of the manuscript. Many thanks to Michaël Dougoud, Chrystel Feller, and Florence Yerly for their constant help during the writing period, and to Rudof Rohr for his help with the figures. A special thanks to Marie Vieli for her beautiful cover painting. Christian Mazza thanks his wife Chantal, along with his children Léna, Emma, Jeanne and Nicolas, for their support and understanding when the process of writing inevitably spilled over into evenings and weekends.

Symbol Description

$\mathbb{N}$	set of natural numbers	$[x]$	the integer part of the real number x
$\mathbb{Z}$	set of integers		
$\mathbb{Z}^d$	set of d-dimensional vectors having integer entries	$\mathbb{E}(X)$	expected value of a random variable X
$\mathbb{R}$	set of real numbers		
$\mathbb{R}^d$	set of d-dimensional vectors having real entries	$\mathrm{Var}(X)$	variance of a random variable X
$\mathbb{C}$	set of complex numbers	i.i.d.	collection of random variables that are independent and with the same law
$\Re(z)$	the real part of the complex number z		

Part I

Dynamics of reaction networks: Markov processes

Chapter 1

Reaction networks: introduction

The central dogma of molecular biology is that the genetic information stored in DNA is used to produce mRNA molecules during transcription, which can then be translated into proteins during translation. The main actors of these two fundamental steps are RNA polymerases and ribosomes. The biochemical processes involved are highly complex, and our present understanding does not permit efficient mathematical modelling. The literature proposes extremely simplified mathematical models which permit us, however, to get insight on cellular processing; see, e.g., [98] where a whole-cell computational model of the life cycle of the human pathogen *Mycoplasma genitalium* provides information on previously unobserved cellular behaviours.

The processes leading to gene expression involve more than 20,000 genes coding for proteins in human cells. Genes are activated by external signals coming from the cell environment, and many genes are also activated from within the cell, e.g., monitoring the degree of folding of proteins. Systems biology aims at describing these intricate and complex processes using notions from electronic, computer science and neural network theory. The main difference with these settings is that the living electronic modules, like proteins (transcription factors), move within cells, and cross structural barriers, e.g., nuclear pores, for example, to reach the DNA, which is in some sense the cell's hard disk. The reader can consult [4] for a clear and fascinating exposition of these various notions, and [120] for a biochemical approach to signalling pathways.

The number of expressed proteins can be small, so that stochastic fluctuations play a major role in the time evolution of these systems, but many proteins are also abundant, especially the enzymes metabolizing carbon sources, which are burnt to yield energy in the form of ATP. The stochastic behaviour of the processes involved in transcription is well documented both in prokaryotes and in eukaryotes; see, e.g., [22], [11], [167], [46], [92], [145], [134], [150] or [143]. Cellular events are, however, well ordered and reproducible, despite the

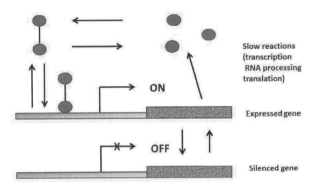

FIGURE 1.1: Modelling of a self-regulated gene with a feedback loop. Regulatory proteins are shown by circles while DNA elements are shown by rectangular boxes, i.e., wide boxes for protein-coding sequences and thin boxes for regulatory sequences. The gene can oscillate between an expressed ON state, where all components of the transcription machinery are bound to the promoter and where RNA polymerase can initiate transcription, and a silent or OFF state. Expression leads to the formation of monomeric proteins in a series of slow processes. The binding of protein dimers to the promoter enhances transcription.

underlying fluctuating and noisy environments. The problem of understanding how cells are able to function in such biochemical noise, and to attenuate or to exploit this intracellular noise, remains one of the most challenging issues of systems biology; see, e.g., [144]. Mathematical modelling provides a natural way for approaching these questions numerically and conceptually, and can also facilitate biological discovery; see, e.g., [98].

1.1   Introduction to modelling: a self-regulated gene

This section introduces reactions modelling a self-regulated gene, which is a building block of many gene regulatory networks. This system contains basic chemical reactions like protein production and degradation. We show in a simple way how such reactions can be modelled mathematically, using birth and death processes.

RNA polymerases begin transcription when regulatory proteins, which are themselves encoded by regulatory genes, are bound to predefined DNA regions located near the target gene, such as promoter regions or operator sites. These regulatory proteins affect the expression of the target gene: they can enhance or prevent gene expression. A gene can be self-regulated, when its own protein enhances or prevents its own expression (positive and negative feedback loops).

Figure 1.1 provides an example where proteins first form dimers, which then bind or react chemically with the promoter region. The gene then controls its own expression through protein dimers. When these bound regulatory molecules have a well defined configuration, RNA polymerase can begin transcription. One says that the gene is ON, denoted by the symbol $\mathcal{O}_1$ later. When the required configuration is not realized, the gene is OFF, denoted by $\mathcal{O}_0$ in what follows. We assume for simplicity that the gene is ON when a dimer is bound and is OFF otherwise.

In reality, protein dimers bind and unbind randomly in time, so that the process can be described mathematically as a stochastic process. We use here the classical modelling framework which assumes that such elementary chemical reactions are described by Markov chains. The feedback loop is modelled by assuming that the **binding rate**, that is, the probability that a protein dimer binds in a small time interval of length h, is proportional to h, with a constant of proportionality depending on the number of proteins n contained in the cell. We hence suppose that the probability of a binding event takes place within a small time interval $(t, t + h)$ is of the order of $g(n)h$ for some function g. For example, for a **positive feedback loop**, one can assume that $g(n)$ is an increasing function of n: the gene product enhances its own production, since high protein copy numbers favour the ON state. The probability to see an unbinding event is likewise modelled as $\kappa(n)h$ for some function κ. If, for example, κ is an increasing function of n, the promoter's ON/OFF transitions are enhanced for high copy numbers, leading to a **negative feedback loop**.

The promoter state thus oscillates randomly between the ON and OFF states, and is described by the relation

$$\mathcal{O}_0 \underset{\kappa(n)}{\overset{g(n)}{\rightleftharpoons}} \mathcal{O}_1. \tag{1.1}$$

This relation provides the transition rates of a two-state **Markov chain**. The function g can be chosen according to the specificity of the setting: we will model these transcription rates using tools from statistical mechanics; see section 5.12. Small regulatory modules of this sort can be found in many gene networks, and the stochastic behaviour of these building blocks thus influences all the other elements. Negative regulation controls the mean expression level, accelerates convergence to steady state, and provides robustness to external perturbations. Positive regulation can lead to multistability, allowing in this way differentiation; see, e.g., [4] for an excellent description of these regulation mechanisms for deterministic models and also [11], [22] or [92] for stochastic ones.

When the promoter is in the ON state, with a bound transcriptional complex, RNA polymerase interacts with the transcriptional machinery, and initiates transcription. The gene is then expressed, leading to an mRNA flux, and to the creation of proteins. One usually does not model all the complex biological processes which form the creation of proteins and influence the speed of transcription, like mRNA degradation, the activation, the sequestration and degradation of transcription factors (TF), but just assume that the probability of production of a new protein in a small time interval $(t, t+h)$ of length $h \approx 0$ is of the order $\mu_1 h$, where the index indicates that the promoter is ON. This models in some way a chemical reaction (the production of a protein) which occurs at rate μ_1, as described by the relation

$$\emptyset \xrightarrow{\mu_1} \mathcal{M}, \tag{1.2}$$

where $\mathcal{M}$ denotes protein monomers. When the promoter is OFF, we assume a basal activity, for some production rate $\mu_0 < \mu_1$, which is represented by the relation

$$\emptyset \xrightarrow{\mu_0} \mathcal{M}. \tag{1.3}$$

These two reactions are summarized through the relation

$$\emptyset \xrightarrow{\mu_l} \mathcal{M}, \ l = 0, 1.$$

Degradation or dilution of proteins is modelled by assuming that the probability that a given protein is degraded during a small time interval of length $h \approx 0$ is of the order νh. This chemical reaction is represented by the relation

$$\mathcal{M} \xrightarrow{\nu} \emptyset. \tag{1.4}$$

Given that a cell contains n proteins, each of them being susceptible to being degraded, the probability that one of these n proteins is degraded is of the order $n\nu h$. This is described by the relation

$$\mathcal{M} \xrightarrow{\nu n} \emptyset. \tag{1.5}$$

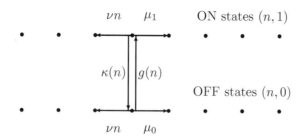

FIGURE 1.2: The Markov chain $(X(t), Y(t))$ evolves on a strip. Nodes like $(n, 0)$ correspond to states for which $X(t) = n$ and $Y(t) = 0$, and form the lower layer associated with the OFF state. Similarly, nodes like $(n, 1)$ of the upper layer are associated with the ON state. Chemical reactions are indicated by directed arrows together with their corresponding transition rates, as given by (1.1)-(1.5).

The time evolution of the state of this self-regulated gene is here described by a pair of time-continuous stochastic process $X(t)$ and $Y(t)$, where $X(t)$ gives the number of proteins present in the cell at time t, and $Y(t)$ takes the values 1 and 0 corresponding to the promoter ON and OFF states. The random process $(X(t), Y(t))$ is modelled in the manner of a Markov chain. We will come to this point in the forthcoming chapters. Figure 1.2 illustrates the fact that this Markov chain evolves on a strip. The idea of modelling reaction networks using time-continuous Markov chains in not new. The author of [38] proposed in 1940 modelling simple irreversible reactions using Markov processes. Most of the works on chemical kinetics were based on *mass action principles*, as formalized by Frost [61], and it was soon observed that fluctuations must be considered seriously for systems involving a small number of molecules. The authors of [37] extended this work to first-order reaction networks. Second-order reactions were also studied using Markov chains in [148], [36] and [125]. Gillespie [67] then provided numerical algorithms for simulating such stochastic processes. The reader can consult [62] or [125] for historical data and results concerning first-order reaction networks.

We study in what follows basic processes which are the building blocks of transcriptional modules. Our approach is based on simple mathematical reasoning, and introduces birth and death processes. More details on such Markov chains will be given in section 2.1. The reader can consult [3] for a nice presentation of the theory, and for interesting examples from biology.

1.2 Birth and death processes to model basic chemical reactions

---

Probability distribution

A real random variable X possess a density function $f(x)$ if

$$P(X \in [a, b]) = \int_a^b f(x)\mathrm{d}x, \quad \text{for any interval } [a, b].$$

The mean value $\mathbb{E}(X)$ of X is defined by

$$\mathbb{E}(X) = \int_{-\infty}^{+\infty} x f(x)\mathrm{d}x,$$

when $\int_{-\infty}^{+\infty} |x| f(x)\mathrm{d}x < \infty$. The variance of X is given by

$$\mathrm{Var}(X) = \int_{-\infty}^{+\infty} (x - \mathbb{E}(X))^2 f(x)\mathrm{d}x,$$

when this integral exists. For discrete random variables taking values in $\mathbb{N}$, the mean is given by

$$\mathbb{E}(X) = \sum_{k \in \mathbb{N}} k P(X = k),$$

when the sum exists, and the variance is

$$\mathrm{Var}(X) = \sum_{k \in \mathbb{N}} (k - \mathbb{E}(X))^2 P(X = k),$$

when $\sum_{k \in \mathbb{N}} k^2 P(X = k) < +\infty$.

1.2.1 Degradation

We illustrate a plausible probabilistic interpretation of the chemical reaction corresponding to protein degradation, as described by the relation (1.5). Suppose that this reaction may happen at discrete times of the form $t = 0, h, 2h, \cdots, kh, \cdots$, for a small time interval $h \approx 0$. Assume that the probability of a degradation in one unit step is given by $p = \nu h$, for some positive parameter or rate $\nu > 0$, with $\nu h < 1$. If time is measured in seconds (resp. in minutes), then ν is measured in the inverse of seconds (Hz) (resp. in the inverse of minutes), to ensure that the probability νh does not depend on the choice of the unit. The number N of steps needed to see such an event is a geometric random variable of parameter p, with (see (1.11)),

$$P(N = k) = (1 - \nu h)^{k-1}\nu h, \ \ k = 1, 2, \cdots.$$

Let $T = Nh$ be the time at which the protein is diluted. One obtains that

$$P(t \leq T < t + h) = (1 - \nu h)^{[t/h]}\nu h,$$

where $[x]$ denotes the integer part of x, that is, the largest integer which is smaller or equal to x. Considering the limit $h \to 0$, T becomes a continuous random variable such that

$$\lim_{h \to 0} P(t < T \leq t + h)/h = \nu e^{-\nu t}. \tag{1.6}$$

T is then distributed according to an exponential distribution of parameter ν:

$$P(t < T \leq t + \mathrm{d}t) = \nu e^{-\nu t}\mathrm{d}t,$$

so that

$$p_t = P(T > t) = e^{-\nu t}.$$

The above reasoning has been performed for a particular protein: let us consider the same problem for a set of n_0 proteins. The probability that a particular protein is not yet degraded at time t is given by p_t, and it follows that the probability $P_n(t)$ that exactly $X(t) = n$ proteins among the n_0 have not been degraded up to time t is given by the binomial distribution

$$P_n(t) = \binom{n_0}{n}e^{-n\nu t}(1 - e^{-\nu t})^{n_0 - n},$$

with

$$E(t) = \mathbb{E}(X(t)) = n_0 p_t \text{ and } V(t) = \mathrm{Var}(X(t)) = n_0 p_t(1 - p_t).$$

The probability $P_n(t)$ solves the following system of differential equations:

$$\frac{\mathrm{d}P_n(t)}{\mathrm{d}t} = \underbrace{\nu(n+1)P_{n+1}(t)}_{\text{degradation of a protein in a set of size } n+1}$$

$$- \underbrace{\nu n P_n(t)}_{\text{degradation of a protein in a set of size } n}, \ n \geq 0.$$

This is the so-called **master equation** or **Kolmogorov forward equation**. It describes mathematically the following balance: the increase of the probability $P_n(t)$ that n proteins in the set of n_0 molecules have not yet been degraded at time t is the balance between the probability that a protein among $n + 1$ is degraded between the moments t and $t + \mathrm{d}t$ minus the probability that a protein among n is degraded during some infinitesimal time interval $(t, t+\mathrm{d}t)$. Let us give some simple arguments. Suppose that the probability that more than one degradation occurs in a small interval is of the order of h^2 when $h \approx 0$ (one can check that this holds true for Markov chains). Since the probability that a particular protein a being degraded is of the order νh, one can focus on the two possible events (the other events having much smaller probabilities)

$$\{X(t) = n + 1 \text{ and } X(t + h) = n\},$$

(a single degradation) and

$$\{X(t) = n \text{ and } X(t + h) = n\},$$

(no degradation), so that

$$
\begin{aligned}
P(X(t + h) = n) &\approx P(X(t + h) = n | X(t) = n + 1)P(X(t) = n + 1) \\
&\quad + P(X(t + h) = n | X(t) = n)P(X(t) = n) \\
&\approx (n + 1)\nu h P(X(t) = n + 1) + (1 - n\nu h)P(X(t) = n),
\end{aligned}
$$

which can be rewritten as

$$P_n(t + h) \approx (n + 1)\nu h P_{n+1}(t) + (1 - n\nu h)P_n(t).$$

Hence,

$$\frac{P_n(t + h) - P_n(t)}{h} \approx (n + 1)\nu P_{n+1}(t) - n\nu P_n(t),$$

when h is small, which is the master equation. The interested reader can consult [147], where many examples from biology are provided.

1.2.2 A basic transcriptional unit

We assume here that the promoter is ON, with a production rate given by some positive constant $\mu > 0$, and a degradation rate $\nu > 0$; see figure 1.3. These reactions are summarised in the following relations:

$$\mathcal{M} \xrightarrow{\nu n} \emptyset, \quad \emptyset \xrightarrow{\mu} \mathcal{M},$$

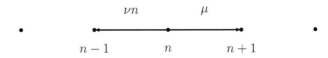

FIGURE 1.3: The basic transcription module. Protein synthesis produces a new protein at rate μ, and one among the n proteins is degraded or diluted at rate νn.

which form the simplest set of chemical reactions modelling protein synthesis, see [139]. Let $X(t)$ be the number of proteins present in the cell at time t, and consider $P_n(t) = P(X(t) = n)$. Proceeding as before, one can guess a master equation of the form

$$\frac{\mathrm{d}P_n(t)}{\mathrm{d}t} = \mu P_{n-1}(t) + \nu(n+1)P_{n+1}(t) - (\mu + \nu n)P_n(t). \qquad (1.7)$$

We provide the way of getting this master equation in section 2.1, but the reader should be able to understand it intuitively, by considering the balance between the various possible events. See [139] for more details.

The Poisson process

When there is no degradation, that is, when $\nu = 0$, the number of proteins $X(t)$ is non-decreasing, and the master equation becomes

$$\frac{\mathrm{d}P_n(t)}{\mathrm{d}t} = \mu P_{n-1}(t) - \mu P_n(t), \qquad (1.8)$$

whose solution is

$$P_n(t) = \frac{(\mu t)^n}{n!}e^{-\mu t}.$$

The random number of proteins present in the cell at time t for the simple reaction scheme

$$\emptyset \xrightarrow{\mu} \mathcal{M}$$

is distributed according to a Poisson distribution of parameter μt, of mean $E(t) = \mathbb{E}(X(t))$ and variance $V(t) = \text{Var}(X(t))$ given by

$$E(t) = V(t) = \mu t.$$

More details on this process are given in section 2.1.

Independence

Two events A and B are independent when

$$P(A \cap B) = P(A)P(B).$$

The conditional probability of the event A given B is

$$P(A|B) = \frac{P(A \cap B)}{P(B)},$$

when $P(B) > 0$. When A and B are independent, $P(A|B) = P(A)$. Two random variables X and Y are independent when

$$P(X \in A; \; Y \in B) = P(X \in A)P(Y \in B),$$

for all events A and B. If, furthermore, $\mathbb{E}(|XY|) < \infty$, then

$$\mathbb{E}(XY) = \mathbb{E}(X)\mathbb{E}(Y).$$

The covariance associated with the random variables X and Y is defined by

$$\begin{aligned} \mathrm{Cov}(X,Y) &= \mathbb{E}((X - \mathbb{E}(X))(Y - \mathbb{E}(Y))) \\ &= \mathbb{E}(XY) - \mathbb{E}(X)\mathbb{E}(Y). \end{aligned}$$

If $\mathrm{Cov}(X,Y) = 0$, X and Y are not correlated. For example, two independent random variables are not correlated. Note that $\mathrm{Var}(X) = \mathrm{Cov}(X,X)$. The variance of a sum of N random variables X_i can be computed using the covariances as follows:

$$\begin{aligned} \mathrm{Var}\left(\sum_{i=1}^{N} X_i\right) &= \sum_{i,\,j=1}^{N} \mathrm{Cov}(X_i, X_j) \\ &= \sum_{i=1}^{N} \mathrm{Var}(X_i) + \sum_{i \neq j} \mathrm{Cov}(X_i, X_j). \end{aligned}$$

When the random variables X_i are independent, it follows that

$$\mathrm{Var}\left(\sum_{i=1}^{N} X_i\right) = \sum_{i=1}^{N} \mathrm{Var}(X_i).$$

The general case

When $\nu \neq 0$, the solution to equation (1.7) can be found using the method of generating functions; see, e.g., [9]. The large time behaviour of the protein number distribution is mathematically described by the **steady state distribution**: one can check that

---

Poisson steady state distribution

$$P_n(\infty) = \lim_{t \to \infty} P_n(t) = \frac{\left(\frac{\mu}{\nu}\right)^n}{n!} e^{-\frac{\mu}{\nu}}. \tag{1.9}$$

This can be seen from example 2.2.3, or using methods of sections 2.2, 3.4 and 13.2. The steady state distribution of the protein number is thus a Poisson distribution of parameter $\lambda = \mu/\nu$. Hence, denoting by $E(\infty)$ and $V(\infty)$ the related steady state mean and variance, we have

$$E(\infty) = V(\infty) = \frac{\mu}{\nu}.$$

One can in fact use the master equation to deduce the following differential equation for $E(t)$:

$$\frac{dE(t)}{dt} = \mu - \nu E(t), \tag{1.10}$$

which is intuitively clear when one thinks about the chemical reactions involved.

Exercise 1.2.1 The time evolution of the number of proteins contained in a cell has been modelled by the master equation (1.7)

$$\frac{dP_n(t)}{dt} = \mu P_{n-1}(t) + \nu(n+1)P_{n+1}(t) - (\mu + \nu n)P_n(t),$$

where $P_n(t)$ denotes the probability of finding n proteins at time t. Use the master equation to deduce that the expected number of proteins at time t, $E(t) = \sum_{n \geq 0} n P_n(t)$, solves the differential equation

$$\frac{dE(t)}{dt} = \mu - \nu E(t),$$

and show that its solution is

$$E(t) = \left(E(0) - \frac{\mu}{\nu}\right)e^{-\nu t} + \frac{\mu}{\nu},$$

which is decreasing when $E(0) > \lambda$ and increasing when $E(0) < \lambda$, and converges toward λ as $t \to \infty$.

Important discrete distributions

A real random variable $N \in \mathbb{N}$, is distributed according to a **Poisson** distribution of parameter $\lambda > 0$ if

$$P(N = k) = \frac{\lambda^k}{k!} \exp(-\lambda), \ k \in \mathbb{N}.$$

The mean and the variance of N are such that

$$\mathbb{E}(N) = \mathrm{Var}(N) = \lambda.$$

Let $0 < p < 1$, and consider an infinite sequence of coin tosses, where the probability of getting a head (resp. a tail) is given by p (resp. $q = 1 - p$). The output of each coin toss is modelled as a binary or **Bernoulli** random variable ε, which takes the values $\varepsilon = 0$ or $\varepsilon = 1$, with probabilities $P(\varepsilon = 1) = p = 1 - P(\varepsilon = 0)$. The mean and the variance are given by $\mathbb{E}(\varepsilon) = p$ and $\mathrm{Var}(\varepsilon) = p(1 - p)$. If we define a success as the event that consists in getting a head, let T be the time of the first success. If the various coin tosses are independent, one obtains that

$$P(T = k) = q^{k-1}p, \ k \geq 1, \tag{1.11}$$

which is the **geometric** distribution of parameter p. One can check that

$$\mathbb{E}(T) = \frac{1}{p}.$$

A random variable S has a **binomial** distribution of parameter $n_0 \in \mathbb{N}$, $n_0 \geq 1$, and $0 < p < 1$ when

$$P(S = k) = \binom{n_0}{k} p^k q^{n_0-k}, \ k = 0, \cdots, n_0,$$

and is denoted by $\mathrm{Bi}(n_0, p)$. The mean and the variance of S are given by

$$\mathbb{E}(S) = n_0 p \text{ and } \mathrm{Var}(S) = n_0 p q.$$

Let $\varepsilon_i, \ i = 1, 2, \cdots$ be a collection of independent Bernoulli random variables of parameter of success p. Then $S_n = \varepsilon_1 + \cdots + \varepsilon_n$ is distributed as a binomial distribution $\mathrm{Bi}(n, p)$.

The exponential distribution

A real random variable $T > 0$ is distributed according to an **exponential** distribution of parameter $\lambda > 0$, denoted by $\mathrm{Exp}(\lambda)$, when

$$P(T > t) = \exp(-\lambda t), \ t > 0.$$

The associated density function is given by

$$f(t) = \lambda \exp(-\lambda t), \ t > 0.$$

The mean of T is given by $\mathbb{E}(T) = \frac{1}{\lambda}$. The exponential function is such that

$$\lim_{n \to \infty} (1 + \frac{x}{n})^n = e^x,$$

where $n \in \mathbb{N}$. Likewise,

$$\lim_{h \to 0} (1 + \nu h)^{[t/h]} = e^{\nu t}.$$

1.2.3 Conversion

We consider here a new kind of reaction, where molecules of type A can be converted into molecules of type B and vice versa, with some forward rate κ_f, and some backward rate κ_r. This kind of chemical reaction appears in most gene networks, modelling biochemical transformations as, for example, configurational changes or enzymatic reactions. This reaction will be represented by the scheme

$$A \xrightarrow{\kappa_f} B, \quad B \xrightarrow{\kappa_r} A. \tag{1.12}$$

The associated deterministic kinetics of chemistry is mathematically modelled by the differential equations

$$\begin{aligned}
\frac{\mathrm{d}[A(t)]}{\mathrm{d}t} &= -\kappa_f[A(t)] + \kappa_r[B(t)], \\
\frac{\mathrm{d}[B(t)]}{\mathrm{d}t} &= \kappa_f[A(t)] - \kappa_r[B(t)],
\end{aligned}$$

where $[A(t)]$ (resp. $[B(t)]$) gives the number or the concentration of molecules of type A (resp. of type B) present in the system at time t, and where κ_f models the probability that a molecule of type A is converted into a molecule of type B per unit time.

The steady state or equilibrium regime describes what happens after a long time and is obtained by taking the large t limit in the above equations. Equilibrium is obtained by setting the derivatives to zero,

$$
\begin{aligned}
0 &= -\kappa_f[A(\infty)] + \kappa_r[B(\infty)], \\
0 &= \kappa_f[A(\infty)] - \kappa_r[B(\infty)],
\end{aligned}
$$

hence

$$
\frac{[B(\infty)]}{[A(\infty)]} = \frac{\kappa_f}{\kappa_r} = K,
$$

where the constant K is the *equilibrium constant* of the reaction.

Cells can contain only a few proteins of specific species, even on the order of 4 or 5, and the dynamics describing the time evolution are noisy and stochastic. Let $X_A(t)$ and $X_B(t)$ be the random numbers of molecules of type A and B present in the system at time t, with $X_A(t) + X_B(t) = N$, $\forall t \geq 0$, since the system conserves the total number of molecules. Using the probabilistic interpretations of the rate constants κ_f and κ_r, one arrives at the master equation

$$
\frac{dP_n(t)}{dt} = \nu_{n+1}P_{n+1}(t) + \mu_{n-1}P_{n-1}(t) - (\nu_n + \mu_n)P_n(t), \qquad (1.13)
$$

where $P_n(t) = P(X_A(t) = n)$, $0 \leq n \leq N$, gives the distributions of the random variables $X_A(t)$,

$$
\nu_n = \kappa_r n \text{ and } \mu_n = \kappa_f(N - n).
$$

The reader can consult [36] and [125] for results concerning such processes. Heuristically, the first term $\nu_{n+1}P_{n+1}(t)$ in the above master equation corresponds to the fact that a type A molecule will be converted at rate κ_r, so that, for the $(n+1)$ molecules of type A, a conversion occurs at rate $(n+1)\kappa_r$. One can furthermore check that $[A(t)]$ and $[B(t)]$ are the expected values of $X_A(t)$ and $X_B(t)$, that is,

$$
[A(t)] = \mathbb{E}(X_A(t)) \text{ and } [B(t)] = \mathbb{E}(X_B(t)),
$$

when all the molecules start from the same distribution; see, e.g., [36] or [125]. Section 3.1 presents networks of interacting species, where chemical reactions like production, degradation and conversion occur, and derives differential equations for the means, variances and covariances associated with the random abundances of species.

Exercise 1.2.2 The reaction which converts type A molecules into type B molecules and vice versa is usually modelled by the deterministic differential equation

$$\frac{\mathrm{d}[A(t)]}{\mathrm{d}t} = -\kappa_f[A(t)] + \kappa_r[B(t)],$$

where $[A(t)]$ and $[B(t)]$ denote the number of type A and B molecules at time t. The reaction scheme (1.12) models a two-state Markov chain $X(t) = (X_A(t), X_B(t))$ giving the number of molecules of both kinds present in the system at time t. Let N denote the total number of molecules of type A or B present in the system at time $t = 0$.

- Assume that there is a single molecule, that is, suppose that $N = 1$, and let

$$q_{AA}(t) = P(X_A(t) = 1 | X_A(0) = 1),$$

and

$$q_{AB}(t) = P(X_A(t) = 0 | X_A(0) = 1),$$

be the law of the Markov chain at time t when the molecule is of type A at time $t = 0$. One can guess the master equation

$$\begin{aligned}
\frac{\mathrm{d}q_{AA}(t)}{\mathrm{d}t} &= q_{AB}(t)\kappa_r - q_{AA}(t)\kappa_f \\
&= (1 - q_{AA}(t))\kappa_r - q_{AA}(t)\kappa_f,
\end{aligned}$$

where $q_{AA}(0) = 1$. Show that

$$q_{AA}(t) = \frac{\kappa_r}{\kappa_r + \kappa_f} + \frac{\kappa_f}{\kappa_r + \kappa_f}e^{-(\kappa_r + \kappa_f)t},$$

so that

$$\lim_{t \to \infty} q_{AA}(t) = \frac{\kappa_r}{\kappa_r + \kappa_f}.$$

- For arbitrary $N \geq 1$, assume that all molecules are of type A at time $t = 0$. Show that $X_A(t)$ is binomial with

$$P(X_A(t) = k) = \binom{N}{k} q_{AA}(t)^k q_{AB}(t)^{N-k}.$$

- Deduce from the preceding point that the steady state distribution of the Markov chain is binomial with

$$P(X_A(\infty) = k) = \binom{N}{k}\left(\frac{\kappa_r}{\kappa_r + \kappa_f}\right)^k\left(\frac{\kappa_f}{\kappa_r + \kappa_f}\right)^{N-k},$$

so that

$$\mathbb{E}(X_A(\infty)) = N\frac{\kappa_r}{\kappa_r + \kappa_f}, \quad \mathbb{E}(X_B(\infty)) = N\frac{\kappa_f}{\kappa_r + \kappa_f},$$

and

$$\frac{\mathbb{E}(X_B(\infty))}{\mathbb{E}(X_A(\infty))} = \frac{\kappa_f}{\kappa_r} = \frac{[B(\infty)]}{[A(\infty)]}.$$

- Show that

$$\frac{\mathrm{d}\mathbb{E}(X_A(t))}{\mathrm{d}t} = -\kappa_f\mathbb{E}(X_A(t)) + \kappa_r\mathbb{E}(X_B(t)).$$

- Generalize the preceding results to the case where the state of each molecule is chosen at random at time $t = 0$ in such a way that the random variables are i.i.d.

1.3   Some results on the self-regulated gene

We give here some basic results concerning the self-regulated gene, as described by the following chemical reactions (see figure 1.4):

$$\mathcal{M} \xrightarrow{\nu(n)} \emptyset, \quad \emptyset \xrightarrow{\mu_l} \mathcal{M}, \; l \in \{0,1\}, \quad \mathcal{O}_0 + \mathcal{M} \underset{\kappa(n)}{\overset{g(n)}{\rightleftarrows}} \mathcal{O}_1. \tag{1.14}$$

As stated previously, the rate functions $g(n)$ and $\kappa(n)$, where n denotes the number of protein monomers, can be described using tools from thermodynamics; see section 5.12. We assume that the production rate is given by μ_1 when the promoter is ON, and by $\mu_0 < \mu_1$ otherwise. If, for example, $\mu_0 = \mu_1$, the system reduces to the basic transcriptional network described in section 1.2.2, with a Poisson steady state distribution for the gene product. Degradations occurs at rate $\nu(n)$ for some function ν, which is often linear in n, with $\nu(n) = \nu n$, for some positive constant ν. The state space is a strip; see figure 1.4.

Let $p_n^0(t) = P(X(t) = n, Y(t) = 0)$ and $p_n^1(t) = P(X(t) = n, Y(t) = 1)$ give the probability of having n proteins at time t when the states of the promoter are $\mathcal{O}_0$ and $\mathcal{O}_1$, respectively. The master equation associated with the reaction scheme (1.14) is

$$\begin{aligned}
\frac{\mathrm{d}p_n^y(t)}{\mathrm{d}t} =\; & \mu_y(p_{n-1}^y(t) - p_n^y(t)) + \nu(n+1)p_{n+1}^y(t) - \nu(n)p_n^y(t) \\
& + (-1)^y(\kappa(n)p_n^1(t) - g(n)p_n^0(t)),
\end{aligned}$$

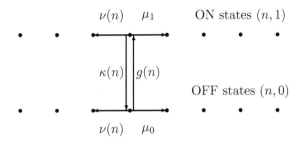

FIGURE 1.4: Illustration of the state space associated with the chemical reactions defined by the rates (1.14).

where $y = 0,\ 1$; see, e.g., [104], which cannot be solved explicitly in general.

Under some assumptions, Markov chain theory provides the existence for $t \gg 1$ of a limiting distribution $\pi_n(y)$, called the steady state distribution, such that

$$\pi_n(y) = \lim_{t \to \infty} P(X(t) = n;\ Y(t) = y),$$

which solves the linear system obtained from the master equation by setting $dp_n^y/dt = 0$:

$$0 = \mu_y(\pi_{n-1}(y) - \pi_n(y)) + \nu(n+1)\pi_{n+1}(y) - \nu(n)\pi_n(y))$$

$$+(-1)^y(\kappa(n)\pi_n(1) - g(n)\pi_n(0)),\ y = 0,\ 1.$$

The authors of [139] solved this equation using generating functions, in the special case where $\mu_0 = 0$, $\mu_1 > 0$, $\nu(n) = \nu n$, and for constant functions g and κ; see also section 1.3.1. Figure 1.5 shows a plot of the empirical frequencies obtained from a stochastic simulation of the Markov chain defined by the relation (1.14). Figure 1.6 provides a comparison between stochastic simulations of the Markov chain associated with the set of reactions given by (1.14) with the exact steady state distribution π, which is obtained using methods developed in [58] and [57], see section A.2, where the stationary distribution

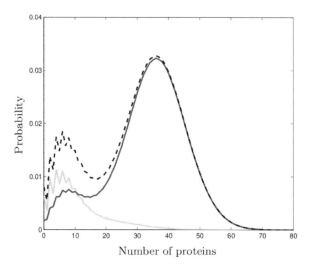

FIGURE 1.5: Simulation of the Markov chain defined by the relation (1.14). The grey line plots the empirical frequencies associated with the OFF states $(n, 0)$. The black line plots the empirical frequencies of the ON states, and the dashed line gives the probabilities $\pi_n = \pi_n(0) + \pi_n(1)$. The shape of this plot reflects the possible bistable behaviour resulting from a positive feedback loop. In this simulation, $g(n) = 0.5n^5 + 150$.

is obtained using transfer matrices.

1.3.1   The case of constant g and κ

We assume here that g and κ are constant functions, $g(n) \equiv g$ and $\kappa(n) \equiv \kappa$. The system is not self-regulated, but the model is important in many biological examples. In most cases, g or κ depends on some inducer concentration v: this happens, for example, in transcription networks where v is the concentration of some transcription factor (TF). Let

$$E(t) = \mathbb{E}(X(t)) = \sum_{n \geq 0} nP(X(t) = n),$$

be the mean gene product at time t,

$$F(t) = \sum_{n \geq 0} nP(X(t) = n, Y(t) = 1),$$

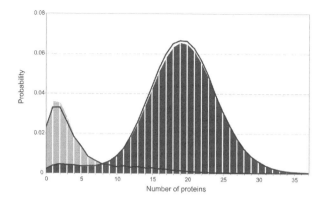

FIGURE 1.6: Comparison of stochastic simulations based on (1.14) with the exact steady state distribution. The grey bars plot $\pi_n(0)$ as a function of n. Similarly, the curve with black bars plots $\pi_n(1)$. Redrawn with permission, after [57], ©2009 by Oxford University Press.

and

$$G(t) = P(Y(t) = 1).$$

The latter gives the probability that the promoter is ON at time t, so that

$$\text{Var}(Y(t)) = G(t)(1 - G(t)),$$

since $Y(t)$ is a Bernoulli random variable. The following differential equations can be obtained by direct computation from the related master equation:

$$\frac{\mathrm{d}F(t)}{\mathrm{d}t} = g\underbrace{(E(t) - F(t))}_{*} + \mu_1 G(t) - F(t)(\kappa + \nu), \qquad (1.15)$$

$$\frac{\mathrm{d}E(t)}{\mathrm{d}t} = \mu_1 G(t) + \mu_0(1 - G(t)) - \nu E(t), \qquad (1.16)$$

$$\frac{\mathrm{d}G(t)}{\mathrm{d}t} = g(1 - G(t)) - \kappa G(t). \qquad (1.17)$$

In the above equation, $(*)$ gives $\sum_{n \geq 0} n P(X(t) = n; Y(t) = 0)$, which is the mean gene product when the promoter is OFF. Note, however, that these relations do not hold in general for nonlinear rate functions; see, e.g., section A.1 or [57].

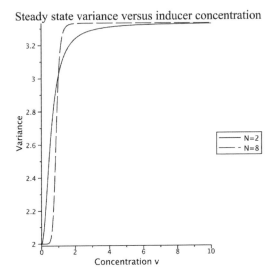

FIGURE 1.7: Steady state variances for a self-regulated gene with $\mu_0 = 2$, $\mu_1 = 4$, $\nu = 1$. $g = g(v)$ does not depend on n, but is a function of some inducer concentration $v \geq 0$, of the form $g(v) = v^N/(1 + v^N)$, while $\kappa = 1$. The plots show the variances for $N = 2$ and $N = 8$.

The self-regulated gene with constant g and κ

The equilibrium or steady state mean gene product is

$$\mathbb{E}(X(\infty)) = E(\infty) = G(\infty)\frac{\mu_1}{\nu} + (1 - G(\infty))\frac{\mu_0}{\nu}, \qquad (1.18)$$

where

$$G(\infty) = \frac{g}{g + \kappa}.$$

The variance of the steady state gene product is

$$\mathrm{Var}(X(\infty)) = \mathbb{E}(X(\infty)) + \frac{\tau_2}{\tau_1 + \tau_2}\frac{(\mu_1 - \mu_0)^2}{\nu^2}\mathrm{Var}(Y(\infty)), \qquad (1.19)$$

where the characteristic times τ_1 and τ_2 are defined by

$$\tau_1 = \frac{1}{\nu} \text{ and } \tau_2 = \frac{1}{g + \kappa},$$

(see, e.g., [57], [137], or [138]).

The interpretation of (1.18) is obtained by observing that, when the promoter is ON (with probability $G(\infty)$), the process evolves as a birth and death process with steady state distribution given by a Poisson distribution of parameter μ_1/ν. The interpretation of the second term is similar. Equation (1.19) shows that the difference between the steady state mean and variance is given by the variance of a Bernoulli random variable (ON/OFF) multiplied by a factor accounting for characteristic times related to protein degradation and promoter fluctuations. Recalling that for Poisson random variables, the mean and the variance are equal, this provides some measure of departure from a Poisson distribution. When $\mu_0 = 0$, the coefficient of variation can be given as

$$CV_N^2 = \frac{\text{Var}(X(\infty))}{\mathbb{E}(X(\infty))^2} = \frac{1}{\mathbb{E}(X(\infty))} + \frac{\tau_2}{\tau_1 + \tau_2} \frac{\text{Var}(Y(\infty))}{\mathbb{E}(Y(\infty))^2},$$

as given in [137]. The above relations yield, moreover, that

$$CV_N^2 = \frac{g + \kappa}{\rho g} + \frac{\nu \kappa}{g(g + \nu + \kappa)},$$

where $\rho = \mu_1/\nu$, and it follows that CV_N^2 is decreasing as a function of g and increasing as a function of κ.

In most gene networks, genes are activated by inducers like transcription factors (see, e.g., section 6.1), and the level of activity of such genes depends on the inducer concentration v. Figure 1.7 shows the plot of the steady state gene product variance as a function of the inducer concentration v. If, for example, the inducer enhances transcription, $g = g(v)$ is an increasing function of the inducer concentration. Typical choices of g are of the form $g(v) = v^N/(1+v^N)$, which models cooperativity; see section 5.12. Usually, N is the number of binding sites where transcription factors interact with DNA; see also the model provided in section 6.1. When $v = 0$, one gets the variance of a Poisson distribution of parameter μ_0/ν, and for large v, the variance is close to μ_1/ν. When N is large enough, the variance is steep as a function of v, switching rapidly from μ_0/ν to μ_1/ν, in the neighbourhood of a critical value v_c.

Exercise 1.3.1 For a self-regulated gene such that both g and κ do not depend on the number of proteins n, establish the differential system (1.15-1.17) and deduce (1.18).

Chapter 2

Continuous-time Markov chains

2.1   Introduction

Many models in science use Markov processes, which form a very rich family of stochastic processes. Let $(X(t))_{t\geq 0}$, be a stochastic process taking its values in a countable space Λ. We can imagine a particle moving randomly in Λ according to certain rules. This process is a time-homogeneous Markov chain when it possesses the following **Markov property**:

$$P(X(t_{n+1}) = x_{n+1}|\ X(0) = x_0,\ X(t_1) = x_1, \cdots,\ X(t_n) = x_n)$$

$$= P(X(t_{n+1} - t_n) = x_{n+1}|\ X(0) = x_n),$$

for every choice of elements $x_k \in \Lambda$, $k = 0, \cdots, n+1$, and $0 \leq t_0 \leq t_1 \leq \cdots \leq t_{n+1}$, and for every $n \geq 1$, when these conditional probabilities are well defined. The **transition probabilities** giving the law of the process are defined by

$$P_{xy}(t) = P(X(t) = y|\ X(0) = x),\ x,\ y \in \Lambda.$$

One can prove that

$$P_{xy}(t) \geq 0,\ \forall t,\ \forall x,\ y \in \Lambda,$$

and that

$$\sum_{y \in \Lambda} P_{xy}(t) = 1,\ \forall t,\ \ \forall x \in \Lambda.$$

The transition probabilities satisfy the so-called *Chapman-Kolmogorov equation*

$$P_{xy}(s+t) = \sum_{z \in \Lambda} P_{xz}(s)P_{zy}(t),\ \forall s,\ t,\ \ \forall x,\ y \in \Lambda.$$

The probability that the particle follows some orbit is given by

$$P(X(0) = i_0, \cdots, X(t_n) = i_n) = \nu(i_0)P_{i_0 i_1}(t_1)P_{i_1 i_2}(t_2 - t_1) \cdots P_{i_{n-1} i_n}(t_n - t_{n-1}),$$

when the initial position is chosen according to a probability measure ν on Λ: $P(X(0) = i_0) = \nu(i_0)$. We will present the main aspects of such random processes. The interested reader can consult [133] and [3], the latter containing many interesting examples from biology.

2.1.1 Birth and death processes

Imagine a particle moving at random on $\Lambda = \mathbb{N}$, jumping to nearest neighbours at random times. Let $(p_i)_{i \geq 0}$ be a sequence of numbers such that $0 \leq p_i \leq 1$, for all i. When the particle is at site i, it can jump either to $i - 1$ with probability $q_i = 1 - p_i$ or to $i + 1$ with probability p_i. Between jumps, the particle waits a random time: let τ_k denote the kth **jump time**, with

$$0 = \tau_0 < \tau_1 < \tau_2 < \cdots < \tau_k < \cdots .$$

The basic interpretation of such a process is that it describes the number of individuals (animals, humans, cells, proteins, chemical complexes) present in a population at time t; a jump of size -1 corresponds to the death of some individual, while a jump of size $+1$ corresponds the birth of an individual. The process satisfies the Markov property under some assumptions: suppose that the waiting times

$$\tau_{k+1} - \tau_k$$

are **independent**. The process will satisfy the Markov property if and only if the random times are exponentially distributed.

Let $(a_i)_{i \geq 0}$ be a sequence of positive real numbers. The random trajectory can be described as follows: when the particle arrives at some site i at time t, it stays there an exponential time $\mathrm{Exp}(a_i^{-1})$, and then chooses its new position by opting for the new site $j = i + 1$ with probability p_i, and for $j = i - 1$ with probability q_i; see figure 2.1. The reader can consult [133] for more details on this construction.

The first natural problem consists in computing the transition functions $P_{ij}(t)$, which are in most cases very difficult to obtain. It turns out that the transition functions satisfy linear differential equations.

2.1.2 The Kolmogorov equation associated with birth and death processes

It is convenient to introduce the following parameters:

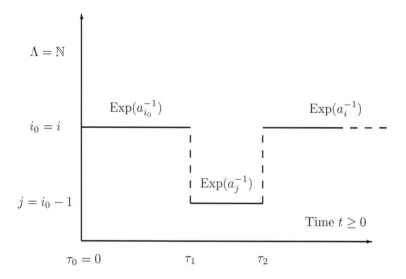

FIGURE 2.1: The Markov chain starts with $X(0) = i_0$. It waits there an exponential time of parameter $a_{i_0}^{-1}$, and then jumps at time τ_1 to the new state $j = i_0 - 1$ with probability q_{i_0}, so that $X(\tau_1) = j$. It then waits an exponential time of parameter a_j^{-1} to jump to the new state $i = j + 1$ with probability p_j, so that $X(\tau_2) = i$.

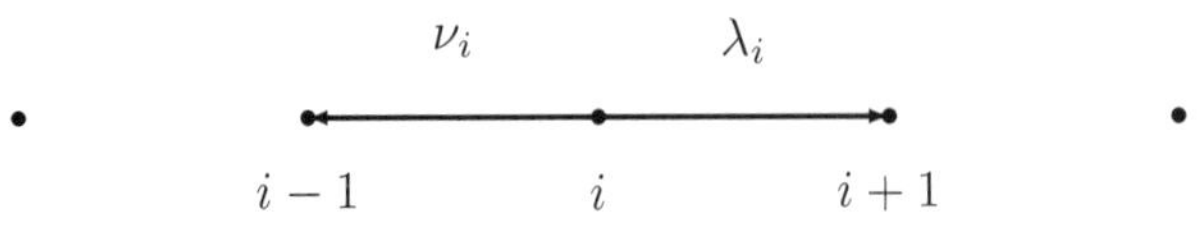

FIGURE 2.2: Nearest neighbours transitions for birth and death processes.

Transition rates of birth and death processes

$$\lambda_i = \frac{p_i}{a_i}, \quad \nu_i = \frac{q_i}{a_i}, \quad p_i + q_i = 1,$$

$$\lambda_i + \nu_i = \frac{1}{a_i}, \quad p_i = \frac{\lambda_i}{\lambda_i + \nu_i}, \quad q_i = \frac{\nu_i}{\lambda_i + \nu_i};$$

see figure 2.2.

The reader can observe that it is equivalent to give the data $(p_i, a_i)_{i \geq 0}$ defining the birth and death process or to use the data $(\lambda_i, \nu_i)_{i \geq 0}$. Moreover, the basic construction shows that, starting in some subset $\Lambda_M = \{0, 1, \cdots, M\} \subset \mathbb{N}$, the process will never leave Λ_M if the probabilities p_i are such that $p_i = 0$, $i \geq M$. This provides a natural way for truncating the process by forcing it to stay in the interval Λ_M.

One can adapt the computations of section 1.2 to obtain the Kolmogorov forward equation or master equation (2.1). The reader can consult [133], where all the mathematical details are presented in a clear way. The books [180] and [3] are excellent references, with many examples from physics and chemistry.

Master equation

Theorem 2.1.1 *Assume that* $\inf_i a_i > 0$. *Then*

$$\frac{\mathrm{d}P_{ij}(t)}{\mathrm{d}t} = \lambda_{j-1}P_{ij-1}(t) + \nu_{j+1}P_{ij+1}(t) - (\lambda_j + \nu_j)P_{ij}(t). \qquad (2.1)$$

The next section deals with the Poisson process, which corresponds to the special case where $a_i \equiv a$, with $p_i \equiv 1$, so that the related process makes only jumps to the right and has the same exponential waiting time on each site $i \in \mathbb{N}$.

2.1.3 The Poisson process

Suppose that $a_i \equiv a > 0$ and that $p_i \equiv 1$. The related process is the **Poisson process**, which makes only jumps of $+1$. These jumps correspond to particular events, the nature of which depends on the modelling framework. Using the above construction, one can check that, conditionally on $\{X_0 = 0\}$,

$$X(t) = \max_k\{T_1 + \cdots + T_k < t\}, \qquad (2.2)$$

where the random variables T_k are i.i.d. $\mathrm{Exp}(\lambda)$, with $\lambda = 1/a$. We will now solve the related master equation. First notice that

$$\lambda_i = \frac{p_i}{a_i} \equiv \lambda, \; \nu_i \equiv 0,$$

so that

$$\frac{\mathrm{d}P_{ij}(t)}{\mathrm{d}t} = \lambda P_{ij-1}(t) - \lambda P_{ij}(t),$$

and

$$\frac{\mathrm{d}P_{ii}(t)}{\mathrm{d}t} = \lambda P_{ii-1}(t) - \lambda P_{ii}(t).$$

We first check that

$$P_{ik}(t) = 0, \; \forall t \geq 0, \quad \text{when } k < i,$$

which is intuitively clear since this process makes only jumps to the right. To see this, observe that

$$\frac{\mathrm{d}P_{i0}(t)}{\mathrm{d}t} = -\lambda P_{i0}(t),$$

with $P_{i0}(0) = 0$, if $i \neq 0$. The general solution of this linear differential equation is $P_{i0}(t) = P_{i0}(0)\exp(-\lambda t)$. But $P_{i0}(0) = 0$ when $i > 0$, so that $P_{i0}(t) = 0$, $\forall t \geq 0$. Next, when $i > 1$,

$$\frac{\mathrm{d}P_{i1}(t)}{\mathrm{d}t} = \lambda P_{i0}(t) - \lambda P_{i1}(t) = -\lambda P_{i1}(t).$$

Using the same argument, we deduce likewise that $P_{i1}(t) \equiv 0$. The general case is obtained in a similar way. On the other hand,

$$\begin{aligned}
\frac{\mathrm{d}P_{ii}(t)}{\mathrm{d}t} &= \lambda P_{ii-1}(t) - \lambda P_{ii}(t) \\
&= -\lambda P_{ii}(t),
\end{aligned}$$

and therefore, using the initial condition $P_{ii}(0) = 1$, one gets that

$$P_{ii}(t) = e^{-\lambda t}.$$

One can check that

$$P_{ii+k}(t) = P(X(t) = i + k \mid X(0) = i) = \frac{(\lambda t)^k}{k!}e^{-\lambda t},$$

showing that the law of the process $P_{ii+k}(t)$, $k \geq 0$, is Poisson of parameter λt. The probabilistic definition of the Poisson processes (2.2) is suitable for finding interesting properties. For example, the Poisson process possess **independent increments**, that is, the numbers of events that occur in disjoint time intervals are independent as random variables. It possesses also **stationary increments**, which means that the probability distribution of increments like $X(t) - X(s)$, $s < t$, depends only on s and t through the length of the time interval $t - s$. For the Poisson process, one has furthermore that

$$P(X(t) - X(s) = k) = \frac{(\lambda(t - s))^k}{k!}e^{-\lambda(t-s)}.$$

Let $Y(t)$ be a unit rate Poisson process ($\lambda = 1$). The new process $Y_\mu(t) = Y(\mu t)$ is again a Poisson process, of rate μ, $\mu > 0$.

2.2　General time-continuous Markov chains

Assume that the state space Λ is finite. The reader can consult [133], where both the finite and countable cases are treated.

The time evolution of this random process $X(t) \in \Lambda$ is defined using transition rates $q_{xy} \geq 0$, x, $y \in \Lambda$, which are encoded in a **generator matrix**

$$Q : \Lambda \times \Lambda \longrightarrow \mathbb{R}, \quad Q = \{q_{xy}, \ x, \ y \in \Lambda\},$$

such that

$$q_{xx} = -\sum_{y \neq x} q_{xy} \text{ and } \sum_{y \in \Lambda} q_{xy} \equiv 0. \tag{2.3}$$

As for birth and death processes, these rates are used to define the infinitesimal transitions of the associated Markov chain: the probability that $X(t+h) = y$ given that $X(t) = x$ is of the order of $q_{xy}h$ for small h, that is,

$$P(X(t+h) = y | X(t) = x) \approx q_{xy}h, \tag{2.4}$$

as $h \approx 0$; see, e.g., [168] or [133]. The transition function

$$P_{xy}(t) = P(X(t) = y | X(0) = x)$$

solves (2.5).

Master equation for general chains

Theorem 2.2.1 *Assume that Λ is finite. Then*

$$\frac{dP_{xy}(t)}{dt} = \sum_{z \neq y} \left(P_{xz}(t) q_{zy} - P_{xy}(t) q_{yz} \right). \tag{2.5}$$

A (line) vector μ is an **invariant measure** if $\mu Q = 0$, that is, if

$$0 = \sum_{y \in \Lambda} \mu(y) q_{yx}, \ \forall x \in \Lambda, \tag{2.6}$$

or, equivalently, if

$$\sum_{y \neq x} \mu(y) q_{yx} = \mu(x) \sum_{y \neq x} q_{xy}, \ \forall x. \tag{2.7}$$

Q is **irreducible** when for any pair of nodes $x \neq y$, there is a path $x_0 = x \rightarrow x_1 \rightarrow x_2 \rightarrow \cdots \rightarrow x_k = y$ such that $q_{x_n x_{n+1}} > 0$, $n = 0, \cdots, k-1$. The natural combinatorial structure associated with a Markov chain is given by a **graph** $\mathcal{G} = (\Lambda, \mathcal{E})$ of node set Λ and of edge set $\mathcal{E}$, which is composed of all possible transitions $e = (x \rightarrow y)$ with $q_{xy} > 0$, $x \neq y$.

When Q is irreducible, one can prove that there is a unique **invariant**

probability measure $\pi = (\pi(x))_{x \in \Lambda}$ satisfying (2.6), such that $\pi(x) > 0$, $\forall x$. π is also known as the **steady state** or stationary measure of the Markov chain. Furthermore, any invariant measure μ is a scalar multiple of π, so that the set of invariant measures is a one-dimensional vector space.

Remark 2.2.2 When the chain is not irreducible, the set of invariant measures satisfying (2.6) is convex, and the extremal elements π_S are associated with the closed, irreducible and positive recurrent subsets S of Λ; see, e.g., [59]. In this case any solution π of (2.6) can be rewritten as a convex linear combination

$$\pi = \sum_S \lambda_S \pi_S \text{ where } \sum_S \lambda_S = 1 \text{ and } \lambda_S \geq 0.$$

Such decompositions will be used in section 13.2, which focuses on mass action kinetics. When the state space is countable and infinite, one defines similarly invariant measures and steady state distributions. In this case, it can happen that no steady state distribution exists even if the underlying graph is irreducible.

Example 2.2.3 Consider a birth and death process such that

$$\lambda_i = 0, \ i \geq M, \ \nu_0 = 0, \ \text{and } \nu_i > 0, \ 1 \leq i \leq M.$$

When the chain starts in the interval $\Lambda = \{0, 1, \cdots, M\}$, it will stay in Λ forever. This defines an irreducible Markov chain on Λ, with a steady state distribution of the form

$$\pi(j) = \frac{\prod_{i=0}^{j-1} \lambda_i \prod_{i=j+1}^{M} \nu_i}{\sum_{j=0}^{M} \prod_{i=0}^{j-1} \lambda_i \prod_{i=j+1}^{M} \nu_i}. \tag{2.8}$$

For example, in the special case of the basic transcriptional unit given in section 1.2.2, where $\lambda_i \equiv \mu$ and $\nu_i \equiv \nu i$, we have seen that the steady-state distribution is Poisson of parameter $\lambda = \mu/\nu$. Let us check what happens for the truncated chain. Equation (2.8) shows that we must compute the products

$$\prod_{i=0}^{j-1} \mu \prod_{i=j+1}^{M} (\nu i) = \mu^j \nu^{M-j} \prod_{i=j+1}^{M} i = \nu^M M! \frac{(\frac{\mu}{\nu})^j}{j!}.$$

Hence, the unique invariant measure is given by

$$\pi(j) = \frac{\frac{\lambda^j}{j!}}{\sum_{j=0}^{M} \frac{\lambda^j}{j!}},$$

which is a Poisson distribution truncated on the set Λ.

It turns out that there is a combinatorial formula giving the steady state distribution π for processes evolving on finite sets Λ. This formula is called the *matrix tree theorem*; see [175] and [24]. We will use it when dealing with chemical kinetics.

We use the notations of [60]: let $W \subset \Lambda$ be a finite subset of Λ. A directed graph g of node set Λ, consisting of a family of arrows $(x \rightarrow y)$, $x, y \in \Lambda$, is called a W-graph if it satisfies the following conditions: (1) $\forall x \in \Lambda \setminus W$, g contains a unique arrow starting at x; (2) g contains no cycles; (3) for $x \in W$, g contains no arrow starting at x. Let $G(W)$ denote the set of all W-graphs. Notice that if W is a singleton $W = \{x\}$, any W-graph g is a directed spanning tree of G pointing to x.

Matrix Tree Theorem

Theorem 2.2.4 *Assume that Λ is finite. Let Q be the generator matrix of an irreducible Markov chain of unique steady state distribution π. Then*

$$\pi(x) = \frac{R(x)}{\sum_{y \in \Lambda} R(y)}, \qquad (2.9)$$

where

$$R(x) = \sum_{g \in G(\{x\})} Q(g) \text{ and } Q(g) = \prod_{(m \rightarrow n) \in g} q_{mn}.$$

When the graph $\mathcal{G}$ supporting the Markov chain is a tree, $G(\{x\})$ contains a single spanning tree pointing to x, $\forall x \in \Lambda$, and formula (2.9) becomes particularly simple, since $R(x)$ consists of a single term, which is a product of transition rates. The reader can see a precise illustration of this fact in formula (2.8), where the numerator of this mathematical expression is just $R(j)$.

2.2.1 Spectral properties*

The linear equation (2.6) shows that any invariant measure μ is a left eigenvector of Q associated with the zero eigenvalue. When the chain is irreducible, we have claimed that the set of invariant measures is a one-dimensional vector space. We will explain in what follows why these properties hold using the classical Perron-Frobenius Theorem. When the state space Λ is finite, let $Z > 0$ be a constant such that $\sup_x(-q_{xx}) = \sup_x \sum_{y \neq x} q_{xy} < Z$, and define the new matrix $\hat{Q} = \{\hat{q}_{xy}, \ x, y \in \Lambda\}$ as

$$\hat{Q} = \mathrm{id} + \frac{1}{Z}Q,$$

with

$$\hat{q}_{xy} = \frac{1}{Z}q_{xy} \geq 0, \ x \neq y,$$

and

$$\hat{q}_{xx} = 1 - \frac{1}{Z}\sum_{y \neq x}q_{xy} \geq 0.$$

This non-negative matrix is **stochastic**, that is, the associated row sums are equal to 1:

$$\sum_{y}\hat{q}_{xy} = (1 - \frac{1}{Z}\sum_{y \neq x}q_{xy}) + \sum_{y \neq x}\frac{1}{Z}q_{xy} = 1, \quad \forall x.$$

Let us denote by λ and $\hat{\lambda}$ the eigenvalues of Q and $\hat{Q}$, which are such that

$$1 + \frac{1}{Z}\lambda = \hat{\lambda}.$$

For any square matrix A, let

$$\rho(A) = \sup\{|\lambda|; \ \lambda \text{ is an eigenvalue of } A\}$$

be the spectral radius of A. A matrix $A = \{a_{xy}, \ x, y \in \Lambda\}$ is non-negative when $a_{xy} \geq 0, \ \forall x, \ y \in \Lambda$, and it is irreducible when, for all pairs $x, \ y \in \Lambda$, there exists a natural number k such that the (i, j) entry of A^k is positive.

Theorem 2.2.5 (Perron-Frobenius) *Let A be an irreducible non-negative square matrix, of spectral radius $r = \rho(A)$. Then,*

- *$r > 0$ and is an eigenvalue of A. This is the so-called Perron-Frobenius eigenvalue of A.*

- *r is a simple eigenvalue of A, that is, both associated left and right eigenspaces are one-dimensional.*

- *A has a left eigenvector associated with r whose components are positive.*

- *A has a right eigenvector associated with r whose components are positive.*

- *The Perron-Frobenius eigenvalue is such that*

$$\min_{i}\sum_{j}a_{ij} \leq r \leq \max_{i}\sum_{j}a_{ij}, \ \forall i. \tag{2.10}$$

The interested reader can consult, e.g., [157] for more information. Coming back to our basic setting, it is easy to check that the stochastic matrix $\hat{Q}$ is irreducible as a non-negative matrix when the generator matrix Q is irreducible. As we have seen, $\hat{Q}$ is stochastic, so that, using (2.10), one obtains that the spectral radius of $\hat{Q}$ is $\rho(\hat{Q}) = 1$. Any eigenvalue $\hat{\lambda} \neq \rho(\hat{Q})$ is such that $|\hat{\lambda}| < \rho(\hat{Q})$, so that $\Re(\hat{\lambda}) < 1$, where $\Re(z)$ is the real part of the complex number z. For such eigenvalues, the related eigenvalue λ has a real part satisfying

$$1 + \frac{1}{Z}\Re(\lambda) = \Re(\hat{\lambda}),$$

so that

$$\Re(\lambda) = Z(\Re(\hat{\lambda} - 1)) < 0.$$

The non-zero eigenvalues of Q thus have negative real parts when Q is irreducible.

Detailed balance equation

An irreducible transition kernel Q of invariant probability measure π is said to be **reversible** when the following *detailed balance* equation is satisfied:

$$\pi(x)q_{xy} \equiv \pi(y)q_{yx}, \quad \forall x \neq y. \tag{2.11}$$

Let Q be an irreducible generator matrix of unique positive invariant probability measure $\pi > 0$. Consider the scalar product

$$\langle f, g \rangle_\pi = \sum_{x \in \Lambda} f(x)g(x)\pi(x),$$

which is defined for functions (or column vectors) $f, g : \Lambda \longrightarrow \mathbb{R}$. Then the generator matrix $Q^* = \{q^*_{xy}, \ x, y \in \Lambda\}$ defined by

$$q^*_{xy} = \frac{\pi(y)q_{yx}}{\pi(x)}, \quad x \neq y,$$

and

$$q^*_{xx} = -\sum_{y \neq x} q^*_{xy},$$

is the algebraic adjoint of Q with respect to the above scalar product, that is, for any pair of functions f and g,

$$\langle Qf, g \rangle_\pi \equiv \langle f, Q^*g \rangle_\pi.$$

A computation shows that $Q^* = Q$ for reversible Q satisfying (2.11), so that such generator matrices are self-adjoint, of real spectrum, and can be diagonalized in an orthonormal basis.

2.2.2   Jump chain and holding times

We describe the basic construction of the random trajectories associated with an arbitrary generator Q.

Definition 2.2.6 *The jump matrix $P = (p_{xy})_{x,y \in \Lambda}$ associated with the generator Q is the (stochastic) matrix defined by*

$$p_{xy} = \frac{q_{xy}}{\sum_{z \neq x} q_{xz}} \quad \text{when } x \neq y \text{ and } \sum_{z \neq x} q_{xz} > 0.$$

Similarly, we set $p_{xx} = 0$ when $\sum_{z \neq x} q_{xz} > 0$, and $p_{xx} = 1$ when $\sum_{z \neq x} q_{xz} = 0$. Let also

$$q(x) = \sum_{y \neq x} q_{xy} = -q_{xx}.$$

P defines a time discrete Markov chain on Λ, of typical trajectory $Y_0, Y_1, \cdots$, with

$$P(Y_{n+1} = y | Y_n = x) = p_{xy},$$

describing the various states visited by the time-continuous Markov chain $X(t)$, $t \geq 0$: when $X(t)$ arrives at some site x at time t, the process stays there for a random time period, which is exponential of parameter $q(x)$, and then chooses its new position y with probability p_{xy}; see figure 2.3. The holding times are independent, and are also independent of the Markov chain Y_k, $k \geq 0$.

This way of defining the random trajectories associated with a Markov chain provides a basic method for simulation, see, e.g., [133]. When adapted to reaction networks, this corresponds to the **Gillespie direct method**; see [65]. For more information on simulations, the reader is invited to consult [66] or [190], where various ways of simulating Markov chains numerically are provided. For an excellent mathematical description of various simulation algorithms of current use in computational biology, see [6]. When the chain is irreducible, the steady state distribution $\tilde{\pi}$ associated with the discrete-time jump chain solves the linear equation

$$\tilde{\pi} = \tilde{\pi} P, \tag{2.12}$$

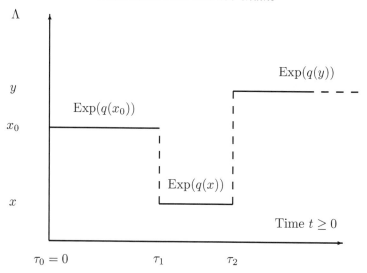

FIGURE 2.3: The Markov chain starts with $X(0) = x_0$. It waits there an exponential time of parameter $q(x_0)$, and then jumps with probability $p_{x_0 x}$ at time τ_1 to the new state x, so that $X(\tau_1) = x$. It then waits an exponential time of parameter $q(x)$ to jump to the new state y, with $X(\tau_2) = y$.

or

$$\sum_y \tilde{\pi}(y) p_{yx} = \tilde{\pi}(x), \ \forall x.$$

π and $\tilde{\pi}$ are related to each other as

$$\tilde{\pi}(x) = \frac{\pi(x) q(x)}{\sum_y \pi(y) q(y)}.$$

This holds true since

$$
\begin{aligned}
\sum_{y \neq x} \tilde{\pi}(y) p_{yx} &= \sum_{y \neq x} \frac{\pi(y) q(y)}{\sum_z \pi(z) q(z)} \frac{q_{yx}}{q(y)} = \sum_{y \neq x} \frac{\pi(y)}{\sum_z \pi(z) q(z)} q_{yx} \\
&= \frac{1}{\sum_z \pi(z) q(z)} \sum_{y \neq x} \pi(y) q_{yx} = \frac{1}{\sum_z \pi(z) q(z)} (-\pi(x) q_{xx}) \\
&= \frac{q(x) \pi(x)}{\sum_z q(z) \pi(z)} = \tilde{\pi}(x).
\end{aligned}
$$

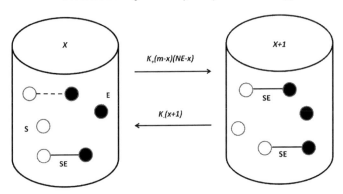

FIGURE 2.4: Transitions associated with the reactions described in (2.14).

2.2.3 Convergence to equilibrium

The large time behaviour of such processes is described by the stationary measure π, solving the equilibrium equation $\pi Q = 0$. We here assume that the state space is countable.

Convergence of irreducible Markov chains to steady state

Theorem 2.2.7 *Let Q be an irreducible generator defined on the countable set Λ, of unique invariant probability measure π. Assume that* $\sup_x \sum_{z \neq x} q_{xz} < +\infty$. *Then*

$$P_{xy}(t) = P(X(t) = y | X(0) = x) \longrightarrow \pi(y), \ t \to \infty. \qquad (2.13)$$

Example 2.2.8 Consider a chemical reaction involving m substrate molecules (S) and N_E enzymes (E). A substrate molecule can bind to an enzyme to form a chemical complex (SE) with rate κ_+. The complex can also fall apart or dissociate at some rate κ_-. These reactions are written schematically as

$$S + E \underset{\kappa_-}{\overset{\kappa_+}{\longleftrightarrow}} SE \qquad (2.14)$$

see figure 2.4. The related stochastic dynamic can be modelled in the manner of a Markov chain $X(t)$, which gives the number of complexes at time t, with $0 \leq X(t) \leq \min\{m, N_E\}$. Let $X(t) = x$: the number of ways of creating a new complex is given by $(m-x)(N_E-x)$. The rate of production of such complexes is hence $(m - x)(N_E - x)\kappa_+$. On the other hand, each of the x complexes has a probability of dissociating during small time intervals, so that the rate of dissociation is $\kappa_- x$. The related master equation describing the time evolution of the probability $P_x(t) = P(X(t) = x)$ is

$$
\frac{dP_{x+1}(t)}{dt} = (m - x)(N_E - x)\kappa_+ P_x(t) + \kappa_-(x + 2)P_{x+2}(t)
$$
$$
-(\kappa_-(x + 1) + \kappa_+(m - (x + 1))(N_E - (x + 1)))P_{x+1}(t).
$$

Let

$$
K = \frac{\kappa_+}{\kappa_-}.
$$

This is a birth and death process of rates given by

$$
\lambda_x = \kappa_+(m - x)(N_E - x) \text{ and } \nu_x = \kappa_- x.
$$

A direct computation shows that the related steady state is

$$
\pi(x) = P_x(\infty) = \frac{m!N_E!K^x}{x!(m - x)!(N_E - x)!} \frac{1}{Z_{m,N_E}}, \tag{2.15}
$$

for a normalization constant

$$
Z_{m,N_E} = \sum_{x \geq 0} \frac{m!N_E!K^x}{x!(m - x)!(N_E - x)!}.
$$

The average steady state number of complexes can be obtained analytically; see [36]. These results will be useful in forthcoming examples from biology, and we therefore give the exact formula. Assume that the number of (SE) complexes at time $t = 0$ is γ, and set $\alpha = m$ and $\beta = N_E$. Let $A(t)$ and $B(t)$ be the number of free substrate and enzyme molecules present in the system at time t. The system is conservative, so that

$$
\alpha - A(t) = \beta - B(t) = X(t) - \gamma.
$$

The steady state mean number of free substrate molecules is (see [36] or [125])

$$
\mathbb{E}(A(\infty)) = K \frac{\alpha + \gamma}{\beta - \alpha + 1} \frac{{}_1F_1(-\alpha - \gamma + 1; \beta - \alpha + 2; -K)}{{}_1F_1(-\alpha - \gamma; \beta - \alpha + 1; -K)},
$$

where ${}_1F_1$ denotes the confluent hypergeometric function. The steady state mean number of substrate-enzyme complexes is, for $\gamma = 0$ and $\beta \geq m$,

$$
\mathbb{E}(X(\infty)) = m(1 - \frac{K}{N_E - m + 1} \frac{{}_1F_1(-m + 1; N_E - m + 2; -K)}{{}_1F_1(-m; N_E - m + 1; -K)}). \tag{2.16}
$$

Exercise 2.2.9 In example 2.2.8, show that the steady state distribution is given by (2.15).

Exercise 2.2.10 Let $X(t)$, $t \geq 0$, denote the size of a population which evolves randomly with the constraint $N_1 \leq X(t) \leq N_2$, $\forall t \geq 0$. Assume that the birth and death rates per individual at time t are given by

$$\lambda = \alpha(N_2 - X(t)) \text{ and } \nu = \beta(X(t) - N_1),$$

for positive parameters α and β, so that $X(t)$ is a birth and death process of rates

$$\lambda_i = \alpha i(N_2 - i) \text{ and } \nu_i = \beta i(i - N_1).$$

Show that the steady state distribution has the form

$$\pi(i) = \frac{1}{Z} \frac{1}{i} \binom{N_2 - N_1}{i - N_1} \left(\frac{\alpha}{\beta}\right)^{i - N_1}, \quad N_1 \leq i \leq N_2,$$

for a normalization constant Z.

Exercise 2.2.11 Let $X(t) \in \mathbb{N}$ be a birth and death process of rates

$$\lambda_i = \lambda i + \mu \text{ and } \nu_i = \nu i.$$

Let

$$E(t) = \sum_{j=1}^{\infty} j P_{ij}(t),$$

be the mean population size at time t when the process starts with $X(0) = i$.

- Show that
$$\frac{dE(t)}{dt} = \mu + (\lambda - \nu)E(t)$$

  with $E(0) = i$.

- Show that
$$E(t) = i + \mu t,$$

  when $\lambda = \nu$, and that

$$E(t) = \frac{\mu}{\lambda - \nu}(e^{(\lambda - \nu)t} - 1) + i e^{(\lambda - \nu)t},$$

  when $\lambda \neq \nu$.

2.3 Some important Markov chains

2.3.1 The Metropolis-Hastings chain

Let $H : \Lambda \longrightarrow \mathbb{R}$ be a function, which plays the role of a potential function in many applied problems. Let μ_β be the Gibbs probability measure

$$\mu_\beta(x) = \frac{\exp(-\beta H(x))}{Z(\beta)}, \qquad (2.17)$$

at inverse temperature $\beta = 1/T > 0$, where the normalization $Z(\beta)$ is the partition function of the system, and is defined by

$$Z(\beta) = \sum_{x \in \Lambda} \exp(-\beta H(x)).$$

Let $\mathcal{M}_h$ be the set of probability measures π on Λ such that

$$\mathbb{E}_\pi(H) = \sum_{x \in \Lambda} \pi(x) H(x) = h.$$

Within the set $\mathcal{M}_h$, the **most disorderly** distribution π maximizes the **entropy**

$$\sum_{x \in \Lambda} \pi(x) \ln(\pi(x)).$$

One can use Lagrange multipliers to deduce that the most disorderly probability in the set $\mathcal{M}_h$ is the Gibbs distribution μ_β for some well chosen $\beta > 0$.

In many applied contexts, one is interested in computing statistical averages of functions $f : \Lambda \longrightarrow \mathbb{R}$ of the form

$$\langle f \rangle_{\mu_\beta} = \mathbb{E}_{\mu_\beta}(f) = \sum_{x \in \Lambda} f(x) \mu_\beta(x).$$

The problems is that $Z(\beta)$ cannot be computed in closed form in general. This causes many strong difficulties, and the idea consists in finding a Markov chain of generator Q_β having μ_β as an invariant probability measure. One then uses this process to get samples $X(t)$ of a law given approximatively by μ_β as t is large; see section 2.2.7. This idea was developed by Metropolis *et al.* [126].

We adopt here the notation $q(x, y)$ instead of q_{xy} for convenience. The idea of the authors of [126] was to consider the so-called *Metropolis chain*: let $Q_0 = (q_0(x, y))_{x,y \in \Lambda}$ be an irreducible and reversible generator of unique stationary measure π_0, that is, $\pi_0(x)q_0(x,y) = \pi_0(y)q_0(y,x)$, when $x \neq y$. The Metropolis chain is defined by the formula

$$q_\beta(x,y) = q_0(x,y)\exp(-\beta(H(y) - H(x))^+), \quad x \neq y, \qquad (2.18)$$

where $(x)^+$ denotes the positive part of x, defined by $(x)^+ = \max\{0, x\}$. The generator Q_0 gives a way of visiting at random the state space Λ. Usually, either this is given by the phenomenon of interest or it is chosen to visit Λ as fast as possible, by respecting locality. Let π_β be the probability on Λ given by

$$\pi_\beta(x) = \frac{\pi_0(x)\exp(-\beta H(x))}{\tilde{Z}(\beta)}, \qquad (2.19)$$

where similarly $\tilde{Z}(\beta) = \sum_{y \in \Lambda} \pi_0(y)\exp(-\beta H(y))$. We claim that this probability measure is the unique invariant distribution of the reversible generator Q_β. The reader can check that π_β satisfies the detailed balance equation

$$\pi_\beta(x)q_\beta(x,y) \equiv \pi_\beta(y)q_\beta(y,x), \quad x \neq y, \qquad (2.20)$$

which yields the result since

$$
\begin{aligned}
\pi_\beta Q_\beta(x) &= \sum_{y \neq x} \pi_\beta(y)q_\beta(y,x) + \pi_\beta(x)q_\beta(x,x) \\
&= \sum_{y \neq x} \pi_\beta(x)q_\beta(x,y) + \pi_\beta(x)q_\beta(x,x) \\
&= \pi_\beta(x)\sum_{y \neq x} q_\beta(x,y) + \pi_\beta(x)q_\beta(x,x) \\
&= -\pi_\beta(x)q_\beta(x,x) + \pi_\beta(x)q_\beta(x,x) = 0,
\end{aligned}
$$

as required. We get thus that $\pi_\beta = \mu_\beta$ when π_0 is constant, that is, when π_0 is the uniform distribution on Λ. This occurs, for example, when Q_0 is symmetric with $q_0(x,y) \equiv q_0(y,x)$.

This method was then generalized by Hastings [80] as follows: Let μ be a probability measure on Λ. The dynamic is again a Markov chain, where one first considers an exploratory transition kernel $q_0(x,y)$, which needs not be reversible (but is of course irreducible). The transition kernel of the Hastings algorithm is then given by

$$q(x,y) = q_0(x,y)\min\{1, \frac{\mu(y)q_0(y,x)}{\mu(x)q_0(x,y)}\}, \quad y \neq x. \qquad (2.21)$$

The reader can check as an exercise that the associated invariant probability measure is precisely μ.

2.3.2 A Metropolis chain on the d-cube*

Let Λ_d be the d-cube

$$\Lambda_d = \{x = (x_1, \cdots, x_d); \ x_i \in \{0,1\}, \ i = 1, \cdots, d\},$$

which is the set of binary vectors of length d, and has size $|\Lambda_d| = 2^d$. For elements x and y of Λ_d, let $\rho(x,y) = \sum_{i=1}^d |x_i - y_i|$ be the Hamming distance between x and y. Let $|x| = \sum_{i=1}^d x_i$ denote the number of ones in x, with $|x| = \rho(x,0)$.

Let Q_0 be the generator given by

$$q_0(x,y) = 1 \text{ when } \rho(x,y) = 1, \text{ and } q_0(x,y) = 0 \text{ when } x \neq y, \ \rho(x,y) > 1.$$

In this case, the related invariant probability measure is the uniform measure with $\pi_0(x) \equiv 1/2^d$. Let $V : \{0, 1, \cdots, d\} \longrightarrow \mathbb{R}$ be a function, and consider the Metropolis chain $X(t) = (X_1(t), \cdots, X_d(t)) \in \Lambda_d$ of exploratory kernel $Q_0 = (q_0(x,y))$, and of potential function $H(x) = V(|x|)$, of unique invariant probability measure

$$\pi_\beta(x) = \frac{\pi_0(x) \exp(-\beta H(x))}{\tilde{Z}(\beta)} = \frac{\exp(-\beta V(|x|))}{\tilde{Z}(\beta)},$$

where

$$\tilde{Z}(\beta) = \sum_{y \in \Lambda_d} \exp(-\beta V(|y|)).$$

The new stochastic process

$$S(t) = |X(t)| = \sum_{i=1}^d X_i(t) \in \tilde{\Lambda}_d = \{0, 1, \cdots, d\},$$

gives the random number of ones composing $X(t)$, or the distance of $X(t)$ to the origin. One can show that $S(t)$, $t \geq 0$, is a Markov chain on $\tilde{\Lambda}_d$, with transition rates given by

$$\tilde{q}_\beta(k, k+1) = \left(1 - \frac{k}{d}\right) \exp(-\beta(V(k+1) - V(k))^+,$$

and

$$\tilde{q}_\beta(k, k-1) = \frac{k}{d} \exp(-\beta(V(k-1) - V(k))^+.$$

Hence, $S(t)$ is again a Metropolis chain on the set $\tilde{\Lambda}_d$. One can check that the unique invariant measure associated with $S(t)$ is of the form

$$\tilde{\pi}_\beta(k) = \frac{\binom{d}{k} \exp(-\beta V(k))}{\sum_{j=0}^d \binom{d}{j} \exp(-\beta V(j))}.$$

These results will be useful when considering models of transcription rates based on thermodynamics.

2.4   Two-time-scale stochastic simulations*

Most biochemical reaction networks contain slow and fast reactions. For example, protein dimerization and the binding of dimers to DNA occur on fast time-scales, on the order of seconds to minutes, while protein synthesis or dilution occurs at relatively slow time-scales of twenty minutes or even longer. Such differences are sometimes designed biologically to achieve specific goals, as, for example, to produce biochemical cycles of almost constant time length in circadian clocks; see, e.g., [55] or [145].

Stochastic simulations of Markov chains associated with such networks can be prohibitively time consuming, because of these time-scale differences: for one slow reaction, one must simulate many fast reactions. Then, common practice consists in assuming a quasi-equilibrium, where the Markov chain associated with the fast reactions runs at steady-state, while the other reactions still run out of equilibrium.

Let $\varepsilon > 0$ be a small parameter, which will be useful for describing fast species; see below.

In what follows, $\eta^\varepsilon(t)$ is a random vector describing the number of molecules of each species present in the cell at time t, and the various possible states taken by complexes involved in biochemical reactions, as, for example, the state of a promoter, which can be in various configurations; see chapter 1. We consider here Markov chains on product spaces of the form

$$\eta^\varepsilon(t) = (\eta_s^\varepsilon(t), \eta_f^\varepsilon(t)) \in \mathcal{E}_s \text{ x } \mathbb{N},$$

where the slow process $\eta_s^\varepsilon(t)$ evolves in some finite space $\mathcal{E}_s = \{1, \cdots, L\}$, and where $\eta_f^\varepsilon(t) \in \mathbb{N}$ visits some subsets of $\mathbb{N}$. Given a slow state $k \in \mathcal{E}_s$, the related fast transitions of the form $(k, u) \to (k, v)$, $u, v \in \mathbb{N}$,

$$(k, u) \xrightarrow{a_{uv}^k/\varepsilon} (k, v),$$

are encoded in a generator of the form A^k/ε. Recall that, according to the basic construction of Markov chains from section 2.2.2, the holding times associated with the fast chain for a given slow state $k \in \mathcal{E}_s$ are exponential of parameter

$q^\varepsilon((k,u)) = \sum_{(k,v),\ v \neq u} a_{uv}^k / \varepsilon$, and therefore the mean holding time is such that $1/q^\varepsilon((k,u)) \approx 0$ when $\varepsilon \approx 0$.

We suppose for simplicity that the state space is finite, and follow [58], where the mathematical results of [192] have been adapted to treat biochemical reactions. The reader can consult the latter to get information on the infinite case, and for time-dependent generators. Assume furthermore that the generator Q^ε of the Markov chain $\eta^\varepsilon(t)$ describing some set of biochemical reactions can be decomposed as

$$Q^\varepsilon = \frac{1}{\varepsilon} A + B, \qquad (2.22)$$

for generators A and B. Following [192], assume that A has the block diagonal form

$$A = \begin{pmatrix} A^1 & 0 & 0 & \cdots & 0 \\ 0 & A^2 & 0 & \cdots & 0 \\ \cdots & \cdots & \cdots & \cdots \\ 0 & 0 & 0 & \cdots & A^L \end{pmatrix},$$

where each block A^k/ε is a generator representing the transition rates of the fast variables given that $\eta_s^\varepsilon = k$. The generator B gives the slow transition rates, and in particular, transitions of the form $((k,u),(j,v))$, where $u,v \in \mathbb{N}$ and $k \neq j \in \mathcal{E}_s$. Following [192], we partition the state space Λ as

$$\Lambda = E_1 \cup E_2 \cup \cdots \cup E_L,$$

where each E_k contains m_k elements, with

$$E_k = \{e_{k1}, e_{k2}, \cdots, e_{km_k}\}, \ k \in \mathcal{E}_s.$$

E_k corresponds to some subset of $\{k\}$ x $\mathbb{N}$, with $k \in \mathcal{E}_s$.

Hypothesis: We suppose that each generator A^k is irreducible with a unique invariant probability measure $\sigma^k = (\sigma^k(e_{k1}), \cdots, \sigma^k(e_{km_k}))$, such that $\sigma^k A^k = 0$.

Following [192], each E_k can be aggregated, and represented by the single state k, corresponding to a particular slow state. The Markov process $\eta^\varepsilon(t)$ of transition kernel Q^ε is then approximated by an *aggregated process* $\bar\eta^\varepsilon(t)$ defined by

$$\bar\eta^\varepsilon(t) = k \text{ if } \eta^\varepsilon(t) \in E_k, \ k = 1, \cdots, L.$$

This process converges in distribution as $\varepsilon \to 0$ toward a Markov process $\eta(t)$ generated by the kernel $Q = (\gamma_{kj})_{k,j \in E_s}$, with

$$\gamma_{kj} = \sum_{u=1}^{m_k} \sum_{v=1}^{m_j} \sigma^k(e_{ku}) B(e_{ku}, e_{jv}), \ k \neq j. \tag{2.23}$$

The reader can see some computations related to quasi-equilibrium in sections A.1 and A.2. The above formula is also valid in the infinite case under some assumptions; see [192] and the following examples.

Example 2.4.1 [A self-regulated gene with a fast promoter] In this example, we consider a self-regulated gene where the transition rates associated with the (ON/OFF) transitions are fast. We modify the relation (1.14) by introducing a small parameter $\varepsilon > 0$:

$$\mathcal{M} \xrightarrow{\nu n} \emptyset, \ \emptyset \xrightarrow{\mu_l} \mathcal{M}, \ l \in \{0,1\}, \ \mathcal{O}_0 + \mathcal{M} \underset{\kappa(n)/\varepsilon}{\overset{g(n)/\varepsilon}{\rightleftharpoons}} \mathcal{O}_1. \tag{2.24}$$

Let us denote by $\eta_s^\varepsilon(t) = X^\varepsilon(t) \in \mathcal{E}_s = \mathbb{N}$ the number of proteins present in the cell at time t, and let $\eta_f^\varepsilon(t) = Y^\varepsilon(t) = 0, 1$ be the promoter state, which correspond to the slow and fast processes, respectively. The slow generator B models production and degradation, as given by the relation

$$\mathcal{M} \xrightarrow{\nu n} \emptyset, \ \emptyset \xrightarrow{\mu_l} \mathcal{M}, \ l \in \{0,1\},$$

while the fast generator A^n, for a given $n \in \mathcal{E}_s$, is

$$A^n = \begin{pmatrix} -g(n) & g(n) \\ \kappa(n) & -\kappa(n) \end{pmatrix}.$$

This is the generator associated with a two-state Markov chain, of unique steady state distribution σ^n such that

$$\sigma^n(0) = \frac{\kappa(n)}{\kappa(n) + g(n)} \text{ and } \sigma^n(1) = \frac{g(n)}{\kappa(n) + g(n)}.$$

The transition rates associated with the quasi-equilibrium process are given by the formula (2.23):

$$\lambda_n = \gamma_{n(n+1)} = \sum_{y_n = 0, \, 1} \sigma^n(y_n) \mu_{y_n} = \sigma^n(0)\mu_0 + \sigma^n(1)\mu_1$$

$$= \frac{\kappa(n)\mu_0 + g(n)\mu_1}{\kappa(n) + g(n)},$$

and

$$\nu_n = \gamma_{n(n-1)} = \sum_{y_n=0,\,1} \sigma^n(y_n)\nu n = \sigma^n(0)\nu n + \sigma^n(1)\nu n = \nu n.$$

The limiting process is thus a birth and death process of rates λ_n and ν_n.

Example 2.4.2 The chemical reaction described in example 2.2.8,

$$S + E \xrightleftharpoons[\kappa_-]{\kappa_+} SE,$$

involves m substrate molecules (S) and N_E enzymes (E). We extend this reaction by adding a reaction modelling the conversion of the complex (SE) into a product (P), of transition rate κ_2, and the production of substrate molecules from a source of rate μ, which models in some way a Poisson source of rate μ. The full set of reactions is described as

$$\emptyset \xrightarrow{\mu} S, \ S + E \xrightleftharpoons[\kappa_-]{\kappa_+} SE \xrightarrow{\kappa_2} P. \tag{2.25}$$

The state space of the Markov chain modelling the time evolution of this reaction scheme is

$$\Lambda = \{(m, x, y); \ m \in \mathbb{N}; \ 0 \le x \le \min\{m, N_E\}, \ y \in \mathbb{N}\},$$

where m, x and y denote the number of substrate molecules, of complexes and of product molecules. We assume here that the reactions associated with complex formation and dissociation are fast. The resulting transition rates are given in table 2.1, where the production and dissociation of a complex (SE) are fast compared to the production of substrate molecules and to the conversion of a complex (SE) to a product (P).

TABLE 2.1: Reactions and rates for the reaction scheme (2.25.)

Name	Transition	Rate
Production (S)	$(m, x, y) \longrightarrow (m+1, x, y)$	μ
Conversion	$(m, x, y) \longrightarrow (m-1, x-1, y+1)$	$\kappa_2 x$
Production of (SE)	$(m, x, y)) \longrightarrow (m, x+1, y)$	$(m-x)(N_E - x)\kappa_+/\varepsilon$
Dissociation of (SE)	$(m, x, y) \longrightarrow (m, x-1, y)$	$x\kappa_-/\varepsilon$

In this example,

$$\mathcal{E}_s = \{(m, y), \ m \in \mathbb{N}; \ y \in \mathbb{N}\},$$

and, for given $(m, y) \in \mathcal{E}_s$,

$$E_{(m,y)} = \{(m, x); \ 0 \leq x \leq \min\{m, N_E\}\}.$$

The generator $A^{(m,y)}$ corresponding to the slow state (m, y) is given by the transition rate $(m - x)(N_E - x)\kappa_+$ for the reaction $(m, x, y)) \longrightarrow (m, x+1, y)$, and by the rate $x\kappa_-$ for the transition $(m, x, y) \longrightarrow (m, x-1, y)$, which are independent of y. This corresponds to the birth and death processes associated with the reaction scheme (2.14), of invariant steady state distribution (2.15). Using the notations of this section, one can write

$$\sigma^{(m,y)}(x) = \frac{m! N_E! K^x}{x!(m-x)!(N_E-x)!} \frac{1}{Z_{m,N_E}},$$

and (2.23) yields

$$\gamma_{kj} = \sum_{u=1}^{m_k} \sum_{v=1}^{m_j} \sigma^k(e_{ku}) B(e_{ku}, e_{jv}), \ k \neq j,$$

so that

$$\gamma_{(m,y)(m+1,y)} = \sum_{0 \leq x \leq \min\{m, N_E\}} \sigma^{(m,y)}(x)\mu = \mu.$$

Likewise,

$$
\begin{aligned}
\gamma_{(m,y)(m-1,y+1)} &= \sum_{0 \leq x \leq \min\{m, N_E\}} \sigma^{(m,y)}(x)\kappa_2 x \\
&= \kappa_2 \sum_{0 \leq x \leq \min\{m, N_E\}} x \frac{m! N_E! K^x}{x!(m-x)!(N_E-x)!} \frac{1}{Z_{m,N_E}} \\
&= \kappa_2 \mathbb{E}(X(\infty));
\end{aligned}
$$

see (2.16).

Part II

Illustrations from systems biology

Chapter 3

First-order chemical reaction networks

3.1 Reaction networks

When a biochemical process contains more than one sort of proteins, molecules or chemical complexes, the dynamics take into account the possible interactions between these various chemical species. There are more than 20,000 genes coding for proteins in human cells, which interact with each other in complicated ways. One actual aim of systems biology consists in finding and understanding these interaction networks. One can propose extremely simplified mathematical models, which are, however, able to reproduce some of the observed phenomenon. The chemical reactions described schematically in (1.14) provide a first basic example of a reaction network, involving production and degradation, as well as a switching mechanism. To go further, we first introduce some basic definitions related to more general reaction networks, and then present mathematical results on linear first-order networks.

The reaction network is composed of M different sorts of chemical species $\mathcal{S} = \{S_1, \cdots, S_M\}$. The **abundance** of species i at time t will be denoted by the random process $X_i(t)$. Let us denote by $X(t)$ the random vector

$$X(t) = (X_1(t),\ X_2(t), \cdots,\ X_M(t)),\ t \geq 0.$$

For a given t, let $P_x(t)$ denote the joint distribution of the random abundances $X_i(t)$, $i = 1, \cdots, M$, where x is the M-dimensional vector

$$x = (x_1, \cdots, x_M) \in \mathbb{N}^M,$$

giving the abundance of each species. The joint distribution is

$$P_x(t) = P(X_1(t) = x_1, \cdots,\ X_M(t) = x_M),$$

for $x_i \in \mathbb{N}$, $i = 1, \cdots, M$. One usually models the time evolution of such processes as time-continuous Markov chains, where the transition rates are defined using the notion of **reaction channels** $\mathcal{R} = \{R_1, \cdots, R_r\}$, and so-called **propensity functions** $W(X) = (W_1(X), \cdots, W_r(X))^T$: given that $X(t) = x$, the probability that reaction R_k occurs in the small time interval $(t, t + h)$ is on the order of $W_k(x)h$. For example, if the reaction R_k takes x to y, the transition rate of the Markov chain is

$$q_{xy} = W_k(x).$$

The **stoichiometric matrix** $A = (a_{ik})$, $1 \leq i \leq M$, $1 \leq k \leq r$ is the matrix where the entries a_{ik} give the change in copy numbers of species S_i when reactions R_k occurs. One can model intricate chemical reactions involving various complexes, which are mathematically viewed as integral combinations of species. We focus here on **first-order reaction networks** where the complexes are reduced to the species themselves.

When the process is an arbitrary birth and death process, of birth rate λ_x and death rate ν_x, $x \in \mathbb{N}$, with $M = 1$ and $r = 2$, the associated stoichiometric matrix and propensity function are given by

$$A = (1, -1),$$

and

$$W(x) = \begin{pmatrix} \lambda_x \\ \nu_x \end{pmatrix}.$$

If the transition rates λ_x and ν_x are affine functions of x, we will see that the mean vector $E(t) = \mathbb{E}(X(t))$ solves the linear differential equation

$$\frac{\mathrm{d}E(t)}{\mathrm{d}t} = AW(E(t)).$$

However, for non-linear rate functions, no simple differential equations can be given in general.

3.2   Linear first-order reaction networks

In this chapter, we focus on first-order reaction networks and on linear rate functions, which are useful when one knows, for example, that some transcription factor (TF) controls in some way some gene without having precise information on this control. Mathematical models of positive and negative control will be provided in section 5.12, they are mostly nonlinear. Linear approximations are interesting since they can be studied analytically, and, in turn, can provide useful insight on the systems. The reader is invited to see [115] for very interesting results concerning the effect of external perturbations on linear gene networks. We present here parts of the results of [62], and focus on Markov chains having transition rates described in table 3.1.

TABLE 3.1: The various types of interactions

Type	Name	Reaction	Rate
I	Production	$\emptyset \xrightarrow{\mu_i} (P_i)$	μ_i
II	Degradation	$(P_i) \xrightarrow{\nu_i x_i} \emptyset$	$x_i \nu_i$
III	Conversion	$(P_i) \xrightarrow{\kappa_{ji} x_i} (P_j)$	$\kappa_{ji} x_i$
IV	Catalytic production	$\emptyset \xrightarrow{\mu_{ij} x_j} (P_i)$	$\mu_{ij} x_j$

Recall that the state space is the set of vectors $x = (x_1, \cdots, x_M)$ where $x_i \in \mathbb{N}$, $i = 1, \cdots, M$ give the abundances of the various chemical species.

Type I and II reactions correspond to degradation and production of molecules, respectively. Reactions represented in type III model conversion where, for example, a molecule of type i is transformed into a molecule of type j: one assumes that each of the x_i molecules of type i can be converted into molecules of type j. This yields the factor x_i in the related transition rate $x_i \kappa_{ji}$. Reactions of type IV model processes where, for example, a molecule of type i can be created when the production of such molecules involves molecules of type j. A typical example is a transcriptional process, where, the gene is active (ON) and hence produce proteins of type i when a TF of type j is bound to the associated promoter.

One of the aims of systems biology consists in understanding the temporal evolution of such systems. This kind of set of chemical reactions is usually treated mathematically using ordinary differential equations (o.d.e.): the number of molecules being large, one can justify o.d.e. using a law of large numbers; see section 12.1.

The linear reaction rates given in table 3.1 define a time-continuous Markov chain as defined in section 2.2: the state space is infinite when the system is open, that is, when the reaction network includes reactions of type I and II. Let Λ denote the set of all M tuples $x = (x_1, \cdots, x_M)$ defining the possible abundances. Type III reactions of rate of the form

$$q_{xy} = x_i \kappa_{ji},$$

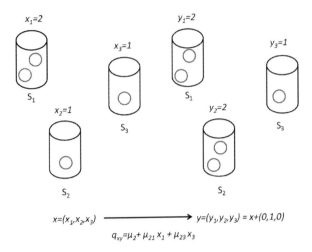

$$x=(x_1,x_2,x_3) \xrightarrow{\hspace{3cm}} y=(y_1,y_2,y_3) = x+(0,1,0)$$

$$q_{xy} = \mu_2 + \mu_{21}\,x_1 + \mu_{23}\,x_3$$

FIGURE 3.1: Illustration of a transition of type IV: a new molecule of type S_2 is created during the small time interval $(t, t+h)$, leading to a transition from $X(t) = x$ to $X(t+h) = y$. The related transition rate is $q_{xy} = \mu_2 + \mu_{21}x_1 + \mu_{23}x_3$.

are associated with transitions like

$$
\begin{aligned}
x \;=\; & (x_1,\cdots,x_{i-1},x_i,x_{i+1},\cdots,x_{j-1},x_j,x_{j+1},\cdots,x_M) \\
& \longrightarrow y = (x_1,\cdots,x_{i-1},x_i-1,x_{i+1},\cdots,x_{j-1},x_j+1,x_{j+1},\cdots,x_M).
\end{aligned}
$$

Type IV reactions model catalytic production, which can be used to model the production of a type i molecule through the transition

$$
\begin{aligned}
x \;=\; & (x_1,\cdots,x_{i-1},x_i,x_{i+1},\cdots,x_M) \\
& \longrightarrow y = (x_1,\cdots,x_{i-1},x_i+1,x_{i+1},\cdots,x_M),
\end{aligned}
$$

of rate

$$q_{xy} = \mu_i + \sum_{j\neq i}\mu_{ij}x_j;$$

see figure 3.1.

3.3 Statistical descriptors for linear rate functions

Consider a set of molecules interacting with each other according to chemical reactions of types I, II, III and IV. One can give a (chemical) master equation describing the temporal evolution of the joint distribution $P_x(t)$, which cannot be solved in closed form in general. It is, however, possible to get information on the means and variances of the random variables $X_i(t)$, and on the mixed moments $\mathbb{E}(X_i(t)X_j(t))$ using generating functions. Let

$$G(t, z) = \sum_{x_i \geq 0} z_1^{x_1} \cdots z_M^{x_M} P_n(t).$$

One can check that

$$E_i(t) = \mathbb{E}(X_i(t)) = \left.\frac{\partial}{\partial z_i} G(t, z)\right|_{z=1},$$

$$V_{kl} = \left.G_{kl}(t, z)\right|_{z=1} = \begin{cases} \mathbb{E}(X_k(t)X_l(t)) & \text{when } l \neq k, \\ \mathbb{E}(X_k(t)^2) - \mathbb{E}(X_k(t)) & \text{when } l = k, \end{cases}$$

where $G_{kl}(t, z)$ denotes the partial derivative of G with respect to the variables z_k and z_l. One then deduces the *partial differential equation*

$$\frac{\partial G(t, z)}{\partial t} = \sum_{i=1}^{M} (z_i - 1)\left(\mu_i G(t, z) + \sum_{j=1}^{M} (\kappa_{ij} + \mu_{ij}z_j - \nu_i\delta_{ij})\frac{\partial G}{\partial z_j}(t, z)\right),$$

which can be solved in some situations; see [62]. It turns out that both the means and mixed moments can be expressed as solutions of ordinary differential equations. Let $K^s = \mathrm{diag}(\mu_i)$, $K^d = \mathrm{diag}(\nu_i)$, $K_{ij}^{cat} = \mu_{ij}$, and

$$K_{ij}^{con} = \begin{cases} \kappa_{ij} & \text{when } i \neq j, \\ -\sum_{k \neq j} \kappa_{ki} & \text{when } i = j. \end{cases}$$

Differential equations for the first and second moments

Let $E(t) = (E_i(t))_{1 \leq i \leq M}$ be the vector containing the expected values of the random variables $X_i(t)$. Then

$$\frac{dE(t)}{dt} = KE(t) + K^s 1 = AW(E(t)), \qquad (3.1)$$

where the matrix K is defined by

$$K = K^{con} + K^{cat} - K^d,$$

and where 1 denotes the M-dimensional vector composed only of ones. The matrix valued function $V(t)$ solves the following continuous-time **Lyapunov equation**

$$\frac{dV(t)}{dt} = KV(t) + V(t)^T K^T + \Gamma(t) + \Gamma(t)^T, \qquad (3.2)$$

(where C^T denotes the transposition of C), where the matrix $\Gamma(t)$ is defined by

$$\Gamma_{ij}(t) = (K_{ij}^{cat} + K_{ii}^s)E_j(t).$$

The mean abundance vector solves thus the linear differential equation (3.1). The properties of such o.d.e. are well-known: we will give the most relevant ones in chapters 9, 10 and 11, and provide some information on the effect of network topology on the dynamics in the sequel.

Let us discuss the existence and uniqueness of solutions to the equations (3.1) and (3.2): the equilibria (see section 10) of (3.1) are obtained by solving the linear system

$$KE(\infty) = -K^s 1, \qquad (3.3)$$

which has a unique solution when $\det(K) \neq 0$. We assume in the sequel that there is a unique equilibrium $E(\infty)$. Proposition 11.2.1 shows that any solution of (3.1) which begins in the vicinity of $E(\infty)$ converges toward $E(\infty)$ when all the eigenvalues of K have negative real parts. In this case, the equilibrium is asymptotically stable; see section 10.7 for a precise definition. Let us denote by $\text{Spec}(K)$ the set of eigenvalues of K. The stability of (3.1) implies that of (3.2); see, e.g., [62] or section B.2.4:

Lemma 3.3.1 *Assume that the spectrum* $\text{Spec}(K)$ *is such that all the eigenvalues* $\lambda \in \text{Spec}(K)$ *have a negative real part. Then both (3.1) and (3.2) have* *unique equilibria $E(\infty)$ and $V(\infty)$ which are stable. Moreover, $V(\infty)$ solves the Lyapunov equation*

$$KV(\infty) + V(\infty)^T K^T + Q(\infty) = 0. \tag{3.4}$$

Criteria ensuring that the real part of the spectrum of K is non-positive are provided in [62]; these results are summarized in the following theorem.

Theorem 3.3.2 *The eigenvalues of K have non-positive real parts when either of the following conditions holds:*

- *The sum of the rates of formation for each species by conversion and catalytic production does not exceed the sum of the rates of loss by conversion reactions and degradation, that is,*

$$\sum_{j \neq i} K_{ij}^{con} + \sum_{j} K_{ij}^{cat} \leq \sum_{j \neq i} K_{ji}^{con} + K_{ii}^{d}.$$

- *The sum of the rates of catalytic formation by each species is less than or equal to the sum of the rates of degradation of that species, that is,*

$$\sum_{j} K_{ji}^{cat} \leq K_{ii}^{d}.$$

Remark 3.3.3 The matrix transpose K^{conT} is the generator of a time-continuous Markov chain (see (2.3)), and therefore, all of its eigenvalues have non-positive real parts. When $K^{cat} = 0$, the eigenvalues of K have hence non-positive real parts, and have negative real parts when $K^d \neq 0$; see section 2.2.1. If, furthermore, $K^s = 0$, the solution is an invariant measure of K^{conT}. When $K^{cat} = 0$, the system belongs to the class of mass action reaction networks (see section 13.1) and the convergence of the o.d.e. (3.1) is given by the defficiency zero theorem 13.1.1; see example 13.1.5.

3.4 Open and closed conversion systems

Assume that only reactions of type III occur so that $K^{cat} = 0 = K^s$. When the chain associated with K^{conT} is irreducible, the solution of (3.1) converges toward the unique stationary distribution; see (2.5) and (2.13). One can thus see the time evolution of the type of a given molecule as a realization of this Markov chain, which moves independently of the others. These dynamics preserve the total number of molecules and the system is closed. When all the molecules have the same initial distribution, let $q_i(t)$ be the probability that a particular molecule has type i at time t, and let $q(t) = (q_i(t))_{1 \leq i \leq M}$ be the related vector. One can then set the following master equation

$$\frac{dq(t)}{dt} = K^{con}q(t), \quad q(t) = e^{K^{con}t}q(0).$$

Using the independence of the molecules, one gets that $P_x(t)$ is multinomial:

$$P_x(t) = \frac{N!}{x_1! \cdots x_M!} q_1(t)^{x_1} \cdots q_M(t)^{x_M},$$

where N denotes the total number of molecules.

When the system is open, that is, when molecules can be degraded and produced, one can find the steady-state solution of the partial differential equations. It turns out that the equilibrium distribution is given by the Poisson distribution

$$P(X_i(\infty) = x_i) = \frac{E_i(\infty)^{x_i}}{x_i!} e^{-E_i(\infty)}.$$

Section 13.2 will focus more deeply on such stationary distributions when dealing with mass action kinetics.

3.5　Illustration: Intrinsic noise in gene regulatory networks

We present a simple model of transcription and translation, and study the effect of feedback loops on the noise structure, assuming linear transition rates. This question will be addressed in more detail in section 12.5 for nonlinear transition rates, using mean field limits and gaussian approximations.

Let $X(t) = (X_1(t), X_2(t))$ denote the number of mRNAs and proteins present in the cell at time t. The authors of [169] provide a mathematical model which takes into account bursts of proteins occur during the synthesis of proteins following loading of ribosomes onto mRNAs. We neglect here such bursts to be as simple as possible, but will come back to this point in section 12.5. The set of chemical reactions is described by the relation

$$\mathcal{P} \xrightarrow{\nu_2 x_2} \emptyset, \quad \mathcal{R} \xrightarrow{\nu_1 x_1} \emptyset,$$

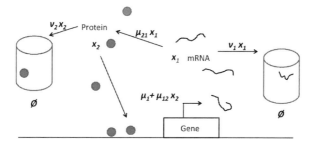

FIGURE 3.2: Transitions associated with the production and the degradation of mRNAs and proteins.

for protein and mRNA degradation, and by

$$\emptyset \xrightarrow{\mu_{21}x_1} \mathcal{P}, \quad \emptyset \xrightarrow{\mu_{12}x_2} \mathcal{R},$$

for the catalytic production of proteins and mRNAs; see figure 3.2. Notice that these two reactions model the possible feedback loops between these two species. Finally, one assumes production from a source only for mRNAs

$$\emptyset \xrightarrow{\mu_1} \mathcal{R},$$

which is associated with transcription, so that $\mu_2 = 0$.

The related stoichiometric matrix is

$$A = \begin{pmatrix} 1 & 0 & -1 & 0 \\ 0 & 1 & 0 & -1 \end{pmatrix}$$

and the propensity function is given by

$$W(x) = \begin{pmatrix} \mu_1 + \mu_{12}x_2 \\ \mu_{21}x_1 \\ \nu_1 x_1 \\ \nu_2 x_2 \end{pmatrix}.$$

One assumes that $\nu_1 > 0$, $\nu_2 > 0$, $\mu_{21} > 0$, and that $\mu_1 > 0$. The authors of [169] assume that $\mu_{12} < 0$ to model a **negative feedback loop**, motivating their computations from steady state perturbations of nonlinear systems. Notice that this might seem cumbersome since for large values of x_2, the transition rate $W_1(x) = \mu_1 + \mu_{12}x_2$ is negative when $\mu_{12} < 0$. The authors of [169] argue that this linear approximation is still valid in the vicinity of the steady state. Nevertheless, we plan to see the effect of the negative feedback loop on the variance. K is given by

$$K = \begin{pmatrix} -\nu_1 & \mu_{12} \\ \mu_{21} & -\nu_2 \end{pmatrix},$$

which has a negative trace. Both eigenvalues have negative real parts when $\det(K) > 0$. This occurs, for example, when $\mu_{12} < 0$ (negative feedback loop). Let $E(t) = \mathbb{E}(X(t)) = (E_1(t), E_2(t))^T$ be the mean of $X(t)$ at time t. Then (3.1) yields that

$$\frac{dE_1(t)}{dt} = \mu_1 + \mu_{12}E_2(t) - \nu_1 E_1(t), \tag{3.5}$$

$$\frac{dE_2(t)}{dt} = \mu_{21}E_1(t) - \nu_2 E_2(t), \tag{3.6}$$

which can be solved explicitly (see the exercises). We here focus on the steady state, and look for the related equilibria (see section 10 for a definition): this means that the long time behaviour is obtained by setting the derivatives to zero:

$$0 = \mu_1 + \mu_{12}E_2(\infty) - \nu_1 E_1(\infty),$$
$$0 = \mu_{21}E_1(\infty) - \nu_2 E_2(\infty).$$

Hence,

$$E_1(\infty) = \frac{\mu_1 \nu_2}{\nu_1 \nu_2 - \mu_{21}\mu_{12}} \quad \text{and} \quad E_2(\infty) = \frac{\mu_1 \mu_{21}}{\nu_1 \nu_2 - \mu_{21}\mu_{12}}. \tag{3.7}$$

One can use (3.4) to deduce the matrix $V(\infty)$, to get that the limiting variances

$$\sigma_1^2 = \lim_{t\to\infty}\text{Var}(X_1(t)) \quad \text{and} \quad \sigma_2^2 = \lim_{t\to\infty}\text{Var}(X_2(t)).$$

are such that

$$\sigma_1^2 = \frac{\nu_1\nu_2(\nu_1 + \nu_2) - \mu_{21}\mu_{12}(\nu_1 - \mu_{12})}{(\nu_1\nu_2 - \mu_{21}\mu_{12})(\nu_1 + \nu_2)}E_1(\infty) \tag{3.8}$$

$$\sigma_2^2 = \frac{\nu_1\nu_2(\nu_1 + \nu_2) + \mu_{21}\nu_2(\nu_1 - \mu_{12})}{(\nu_1\nu_2 - \mu_{21}\mu_{12})(\nu_1 + \nu_2)}E_2(\infty). \tag{3.9}$$

Suppose that there is no feedback from the protein on mRNA production, that is, assume that $\mu_{12} = 0$. Then

$$E_1(\infty) = \frac{\mu_1}{\nu_1} = \sigma_1^2.$$

This is natural since, in this particular situation, the process $X_1(t)$ is independent of $X_2(t)$ and evolves as a simple birth and death process of birth rate μ_1 and death rate ν_1, with a Poisson steady state of parameter $\lambda = \frac{\mu_1}{\nu_1}$ (see (1.9)). One can check that σ_2 is increasing as a function of μ_{12} for $\mu_{12} < \nu_1\nu_2/\mu_{21}$. In this case, the above formula for σ_2^2 shows that such **negative feedback loops can reduce the variance of the intrinsic noise**; see, e.g., [137], [173] or [113].

Exercise 3.5.1 • Solve the linear differential system defined by (3.5) and (3.6), and compute the limiting values of $E_1(t)$ and $E_2(t)$ as $t \to \infty$.

• Use (3.4) to find the matrix $V(\infty)$, and then deduce the variances as given by (3.8) and (3.9).

• Show that σ_2^2 is an increasing function of μ_{12} when $\mu_{12} < \nu_1\nu_2/\mu_{21}$.

Chapter 4

Biochemical pathways

4.1   Stochastic fluctuations in metabolic pathways

The metabolism converts biological material into energy or produces the building blocks needed to construct biological structures, maintain cells or carry out various cellular functions; see ,e.g., [135] for a systems biology approach. It is impossible to give a simple overview of the properties of metabolic pathways; here, we illustrate briefly very simple models which aim at showing how one can get insight on such complicated processes using mathematical modelling. Deterministic models are of current use to study complex metabolic networks; see, e.g., [154], [141], [82] or [166], and the references therein. We focus here on examples of stochastic models.

When chemical compounds like metabolites are present in high copy numbers, the related chemical kinetics can be described macroscopically, neglecting stochastic fluctuations. This approach can be misleading in cells where biochemical pathways can involve chemical species of low abundance. We follow here [44] and [114]. The authors of [114] present a well known *E. coli* pathway, where an incoming flux of substrate molecules is converted through enzymatic reactions into a product flux. In this example, *tryptophan biosynthesis*, an incoming flux of chorismate, is converted by six reactions into a tryptophan flux; see, e.g., [127]. Their approach uses the mathematical models developed in examples 2.2.8 and 2.4.2, where the generic chemical reaction is given by the relation (2.25):

$$\emptyset \xrightarrow{\mu} S, \ S + E \underset{\kappa_-}{\overset{\kappa_+}{\longleftrightarrow}} SE \xrightarrow{\kappa_2} P.$$

Example 2.4.2 assumes fast equilibration between the substrate and the enzyme. In this limit, the process reduces to a birth and death process of rates

$$\lambda_m = \mu,$$

and

$$\nu_m = \kappa_2 \mathbb{E}(X(\infty))$$

(see (2.16)) when $m \le N_E$, where we recall that m and N_E denote the number of substrate and enzyme molecules. The authors of [44] and [114] focus a large product limit $K = \kappa_+/\kappa_- \gg 1$ to simplify the above transition rates, and obtain that

$$\nu_m = \kappa_2 \frac{m}{m + (K - N_E - 1)}, \quad K \to \infty, \tag{4.1}$$

which is the so-called **Michaelis Menten** law. A direct computation then shows that the steady state distribution is of the form

$$\pi(m) = \binom{m + K + N_E - 1}{m}(1 - z)^{K + N_E m}, \tag{4.2}$$

where $z = \mu/\nu_{\max}$.

The authors of [114] consider a set of M substrate types $S_1, S_2, \cdots, S_M$. The species S_1 is produced as a Poisson process of rate μ, and the evolution of the abundance of S_1 molecules is described by the reaction scheme (2.25). The reaction associated with species S_i, for $2 \le i \le M$, is

$$S_i + E_i \underset{\kappa_-^i}{\overset{\kappa_+^i}{\longleftrightarrow}} SE_i \overset{\kappa_2^i}{\longrightarrow} S_{i+1}, \tag{4.3}$$

where E_i denotes the enzyme associated with the ith reaction. These authors then observe that this set of metabolic reactions can be seen as a **particle system**. The abundance of each species, $X_i \in \mathbb{N}$, fluctuates randomly as a Markov chain $X(t) = (X_1(t), \cdots, X_M(t))$ of state space

$$\Lambda = \{x = (x_1, \cdots, x_M); \ x_i \in \mathbb{N}\}.$$

Biochemical pathways are usually very intricate, and metabolic networks should be described as directed graphs, of node set $S = \{S_1, \cdots, S_M\}$. We hence assume a graph structure $\mathcal{G} = (\mathcal{S}, \mathcal{E})$ of node set $\mathcal{S}$ and (directed) edge set $\mathcal{E}$. Edges are generically denoted by $e = (S_i \to S_j)$, meaning that a substrate molecule of species S_i can be converted into a substrate molecule of type S_j, at rate κ_{ji}.

Let e_i denote the ith unit vector of $\mathbb{R}^M$, that is, the vector having all components equal to 0 except the ith one, which is equal to 1. The transitions of the particle system are of the form

$$(x \to x - e_i + e_j) \text{ when } e = (S_i \to S_j) \in \mathcal{E},$$

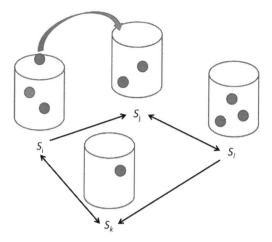

FIGURE 4.1: The directed edges of the graph $\mathcal{G}$ are represented by arrows. A molecule of type S_i is being converted (or transported) into a type S_j molecule.

meaning that a particle of species S_i has been converted into a molecule of type S_j, at rate

$$q_{x,x-e_i+e_j} = \kappa_{ji}\nu_{x_i}.$$

These kinds of mass-transport particle systems are well known in statistical physics and in probability theory, and are called **zero-range processes**; see [107]. In other words, particles move randomly according to the following rules: a particle located at site i (or of type S_i) can move toward one of its nearest neighbours j with $(S_i \to S_j) \in \mathcal{E}$ at rate $\kappa_{ji}\nu_{x_i}$, which depends on the number of molecules of type S_i.

The probabilistic literature considers mostly hydrodynamical limits where the number of sites $M \to \infty$ and the number of particles is scaled to a fixed density. One then observes condensation phenomena; see [73]. In biochemical pathways, the number of types is not too large, so that one should consider different approximations, for example, assuming only that the number of molecules is large enough.

Let $P_x(t)$ be the law of the particle system, with

$$P_x(t) = P(X_1(t) = x_1, \cdots, X_M(t) = x_M),$$

where $x_i \in \mathbb{N}$. The master equation is

$$\frac{dP_x(t)}{dt} = \sum_{(S_i \to S_j) \in \mathcal{E}} \left(P_{x-e_j+e_i}(t) q_{x-e_j+e_i, n} - P_x(t) q_{x, x-e_i+e_j} \right)$$

$$+ \sum_i P_{x-e_i}(t)\mu_i - \sum_j P_x(t)\mu_j.$$

One can first look for the steady state distribution $\pi(x_1, \cdots, x_M)$ by setting the derivatives to 0. The literature provides criteria ensuring that this probability distribution factorises as a product

$$\pi(x_1, \cdots, x_M) = \pi_1(x_1) \cdots \pi_M(x_M), \tag{4.4}$$

(see chapter 13) where the factors are given by the marginal laws (4.2). When (4.4) is satisfied, and when no conservation law restricts the possible values of the x_i (see section 13), the steady state random variables $X_i(\infty)$ are independent, so that the random fluctuations of some species have no effect on the other types. This conclusion is apparently different from the conclusions obtained for some gene networks; see, e.g., [137].

Regulation of such networks can be obtained by modifying enzyme concentrations and using feedback loops; see [135]. The connectivity of typical metabolic networks is such that, on the average, more than five metabolites are located one step away from a given metabolite; see, e.g., [183]. We will provide conditions ensuring that the stationary measure is a product measure in section 13.2. The authors of [114] provide interesting simulations where one can notice that steady state distributions are well approximated by such product measures in a large variety of graphs.

Some interesting biological conclusions can be derived from this decorrelation: the steady state statistical fluctuations of some substrate S_i only depend on the concentration of enzyme E_{i-1}. This property allows the regulation of toxic intermediates by fine tuning the related enzymes. Being independent at steady state, the properties of each node can be modified without altering the nature of the others. These facts might be designed by evolution to allow adaptation to changing environments without modifying the fluctuations at other nodes. Moreover, according to this model, steady state fluctuations do not give information on the pathway structure (see, e.g., [163] for a bioinformatical confirmation of this fact). Hence, pathway structures should be studied using more mechanistic methods; see, e.g., [135] for a detailed presentation.

4.2 Signalling networks

Cells receive information from their environment, and, in turn, respond in a way that is coded by their genes and epigenetic factors. Cells are able to respond to many chemical and physical agents which can induce transitory or permanent changes in cells. These signalling molecules bind to protein receptors, which interact with special proteins in the cytoplasmic or plasma membrane. The latter then transduce (or send) the signal to deeper levels within the cell. Protein kinases and protein phosphatases mediate a significant part of the signal transduction in eukaryotic cells. The human kinome contains more than 500 types of protein kinase (see, e.g., [118]) and approximatively 150 types of protein phosphatase. These pathways are designed to elicit a cellular response like the activation of transcription factors in response to external signals, and thus increase the expression of some target genes, producing in this way mRNA flux; see, e.g., [120] for a nice exposition of cellular processing, from the point of view of systems biology. The network structures associated with these protein or signalling networks are similar to the topologies observed in metabolic networks, and contain positive and negative feedback loops; see, e.g., [135]. Cellular processing units are designed and work like electronic circuits or neural networks; see, e.g., chapter 6 of [4], where such pathways are studied using tools from neural network theory. A basic difference is that the living processing units involved can move and diffuse inside the cell. It is difficult to give a general overview of the various existing topologies. The reader can consult, among others, [52], [191], [13], [177], [116], [53] and [151] to get ideas on known network structures.

We present here a mathematical model of [83] which focuses mainly on linear kinase-phosphatase cascades, and describes their sequential activation when an external stimulation induces the activation of several downstream protein kinases, and ends with the phosphorylation of the last kinase. This can elicit a cellular response to the input signal. This signalling pathway then ends under the action of phosphatase.

We begin by proposing a stochastic model, taking inspiration from the existing literature, and focus next on the model of [83]: the first kinase is activated by some external signal $R(t)$, $t \geq 0$. Let $Y_1(t)$ be a Bernoulli random variable describing the activity of the first kinase at time t, with $Y_1(t) = 1$ when it is active, or phosphorylated, and $Y_1(t) = 0$ otherwise. The related dynamic might be described by a time non-homogeneous two-state Markov chain. The transition rate from the OFF state to the ON state is proportional to the signal amplitude, of the form $\tilde{\alpha}_1 R(t)$. The reverse transition is described by a constant rate β_1. This reaction is then modelled by the relation

$$\mathcal{O}_0^1 \underset{\beta_1}{\overset{\tilde{\alpha}_1 R(t)}{\longleftrightarrow}} \mathcal{O}_1^1. \tag{4.5}$$

For the remaining kinases of type $i \geq 2$, let $Y_i(t) = 0, 1$ denote the activity of the ith kinase at time t. In a linear cascade, the state of the ith kinase depends on the state of the $(i-1)$th kinase (see figure 4.2): for example, MAPK pathways which respond to pheromones, a scaffold protein tethers the kinases, perhaps to avoid cross-talks between pathways; see, e.g., [120] or [151]. Hence, one can assume that there is a direct link between consecutive kinases. The rate of transition from the OFF state to the ON state is modelled as $\tilde{\alpha}_i Y_{i-1}(t)$. The reverse transition is also given by a constant rate β_i. This reaction is summarized by the relation

$$\mathcal{O}_0^i \underset{\beta_i}{\overset{\tilde{\alpha}_i Y_{i-1}}{\longleftrightarrow}} \mathcal{O}_1^i; \tag{4.6}$$

see figure 4.2. The state of the system at time t is described by the random binary vector $Y(t) = (Y_1(t), \cdots, Y_M(t))$. Let $E_i(t) = \mathbb{E}(Y_i(t)) = P(Y_i(t) = 1)$. The related master equation yields that

$$\frac{dE_i(t)}{dt} = \tilde{\alpha}_i \mathbb{E}((1 - Y_i(t))Y_{i-1}(t)) - \beta_i E_i(t),$$

when $i \geq 2$. Due to statistical correlations,

$$\mathbb{E}((1 - Y_i(t))Y_{i-1}(t)) \neq \mathbb{E}((1 - Y_i(t)))\mathbb{E}(Y_{i-1}(t)) = (1 - E_i(t))E_{i-1}(t),$$

in general. If these random variables are not correlated, one obtains the o.d.e.

$$\frac{dE_i(t)}{dt} = \tilde{\alpha}_i(1 - E_i(t))E_{i-1}(t) - \beta_i E_i(t).$$

The authors of [83] study this last o.d.e., using variables $X_i(t)$, describing kinase abundances: let C_i denote the total number of type i kinases, which can be active or not. Their model is given by the set of differential equations

$$\frac{dX_1(t)}{dt} = \tilde{\alpha}_1 R(t)(C_1 - X_1(t)) - \beta_1 X_1(t),$$

$$\frac{dX_i(t)}{dt} = \tilde{\alpha}_i X_{i-1}(t)(C_i - X_i(t)) - \beta_i X_i(t), \ i \geq 2.$$

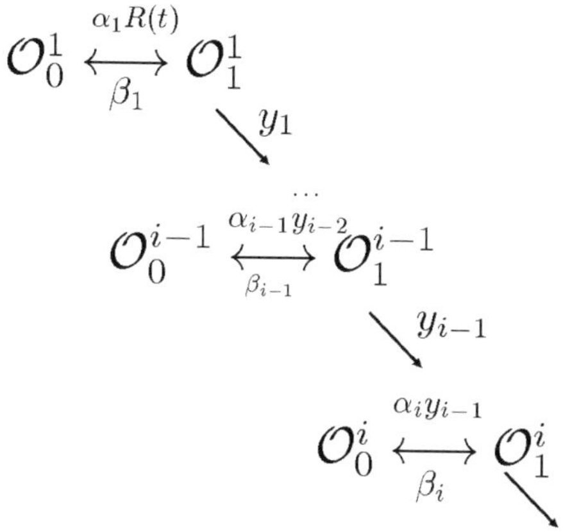

$$\mathcal{O}_0^1 \underset{\beta_1}{\overset{\alpha_1 R(t)}{\longleftrightarrow}} \mathcal{O}_1^1$$

$$\searrow y_1$$

$$\cdots$$

$$\mathcal{O}_0^{i-1} \underset{\beta_{i-1}}{\overset{\alpha_{i-1} y_{i-2}}{\longleftrightarrow}} \mathcal{O}_1^{i-1}$$

$$\searrow y_{i-1}$$

$$\mathcal{O}_0^{i} \underset{\beta_i}{\overset{\alpha_i y_{i-1}}{\longleftrightarrow}} \mathcal{O}_1^{i}$$

$$\searrow$$

FIGURE 4.2: The signalling cascade. The phosphorylation rate of the first kinase depends on the external signal $R(t)$. $\mathcal{O}_0^i$ denotes the OFF state, and $\mathcal{O}_1^i$ the ON state.

The **signalling time** τ_i is defined to be the average time needed to activate a kinase of type i. The formal definition of τ_i makes use of the density function

$$f_i(t) = \frac{X_i(t)}{\int_0^\infty X_i(s)\mathrm{d}s}, t > 0.$$

Let $T_i > 0$ be a random variable of density f_i. The signalling time τ_i is the expected value of T_i, that is,

$$\tau_i = \mathbb{E}(T_i) = \int_0^\infty t f_i(t)\mathrm{d}t.$$

The **signal duration** is the related standard deviation

$$\sigma_i = \sqrt{\mathrm{Var}(T_i)} = \sqrt{\mathbb{E}(T_i^2) - (\mathbb{E}(T_i))^2},$$

where we recall that

$$\mathbb{E}(T_i^2) = \int_0^\infty t^2 f_i(t)\mathrm{d}t.$$

One more characteristic that can be of interest is the **signal amplitude** A_i,

$$A_i = \frac{\int_0^\infty X_i(s)\mathrm{d}s}{2\sigma_i},$$

which is the height of a rectangle of length $2\sigma_i$ of area $l_i = \int_0^\infty X_i(s)\mathrm{d}s$.

Weakly activated pathways

For weakly activated pathways such that $X_i(t)/C_i \approx 0$ and $X_i(0) = 0$, $\forall i$, and for exponentially decaying input signals of the form $R(t) = R(0) \exp(-\lambda t)$, $\lambda > 0$, the authors of [83] observed that

$$\tau_M = \frac{1}{\lambda} + \sum_{i=1}^{M} \frac{1}{\beta_i}, \tag{4.7}$$

which does not depend on the phosphorylation rate α_i. Moreover, all the phosphatases have the same effect on the signalling time, regardless of their position in the pathway. They also observed the same phenomenon for the signal duration,

$$\sigma_M = \sqrt{\frac{1}{\lambda^2} + \sum_{i=1}^{M} \frac{1}{\beta_i^2}}. \tag{4.8}$$

In contrast, the signal amplitude depends on all the pathway parameters

$$A_M = \frac{R(0) \prod_{i=1}^{M} \frac{\alpha_i}{\beta_i}}{2\sqrt{1 + \lambda^2 \sum_{i=1}^{M} \frac{1}{\beta_i^2}}}, \tag{4.9}$$

where we set

$$\alpha_i = C_i \tilde{\alpha}_i.$$

The signal can be amplified, that is, $A_{i-1} < A_i$ when

$$\beta_i < \alpha_i \sqrt{1 - \frac{1}{\alpha_i^2 \sigma_{i-1}^2}},$$

so that there is some amplification when the dephosphorylation rate β_i is small relative to α_i.

Formulas (4.7) and (4.8) show that both the signalling time τ_M and the signal duration σ_M increase as functions of the cascade length M, so that, at a first sight, it might seem plausible that longer signalling cascades lead to larger signalling times. On the other hand, the signal amplitude (4.9) can also be increasing as a function of M: in this case, the amplitude can become larger with long signalling cascades, and one can thus achieve a given level of amplification using a few steps of large amplitude. Simulations performed by the authors of [83] show the surprising fact that one can find parameter regimes where long signalling cascades lead to faster cascades. They conjecture the existence of an optimal cascade length resulting in a minimum for signalling time and duration.

These computations have been generalized to a large class of input signals $R(t)$ in [29], where mathematical techniques from control theory have been used. The above conjecture is true under very general conditions. Weakly activated cascades can therefore play the role of amplifiers, as in electronic circuits where such modules are currently used.

Strongly activated pathways

For strongly activated cascades, the abundances $X_i(t)$ saturate quickly, so that the authors of [83] assumed that

$$\frac{\mathrm{d}X_i(t)}{\mathrm{d}t} \approx 0.$$

The equilibrium is described by the equation

$$\alpha_i X_{i-1}(t)(1 - \frac{X_i(t)}{C_i}) = \beta_i X_i(t),$$

so that

$$X_i = \frac{X_{i-1}}{\frac{\beta_i}{\alpha_i} + \frac{X_{i-1}}{C_i}}. \tag{4.10}$$

There is some amplification with $X_{i-1} < X_i$ when

$$X_{i-1} < C_i(1 - \frac{\beta_i}{\alpha_i}).$$

The condition $\beta_i < \alpha_i$ is necessary for amplification, but is not sufficient to ensure amplification (X_{i-1} must also be smaller than C_i). The authors of [83] then deduced that signal amplification is less pronounced for strongly activated signalling cascades.

These biological conclusions have been obtained using the deterministic approach, which neglects stochastic fluctuations. It might be of interest to compute these quantities for the stochastic system. Similar models were presented recently to study amplification properties of the mammalian mitogen-activated protein kinase (MAPK) pathway; see [165] and the references therein. These authors used a mathematical model of [153] to show that three-tiered kinase amplifiers combined with negative feedback loops possess the same properties as negative feedback amplifiers used in electronic circuits; see, e.g., [21] or [136]. These modules are used in engineering for their ability to provide robustness and output stabilization, among other desirable properties. This is a good example which shows how systems biology questions can be approached using methods developed in mathematics, control theory and physics. It also shows that signalling cascades can be seen as living electronic modules; see, e.g., [120].

The next natural question consists in understanding, for example, how the last kinase transduces the signal spatially toward the nucleus. Various scenarios have been envisaged; see, e.g., [119] and [117], where one suspects that kinases are transported or move randomly by diffusion to reach the nucleus. It has been proven that simple diffusion can not ensure signal transduction; see, e.g., [119]. This is quite an open field of research at the present time, and interesting mathematical models exist which are based on reaction-diffusion processes; see, e.g., [162], [117] or [72].

Exercise 4.2.1 The differential system associated with weakly activated linear activation cascades is

$$\frac{dX_1(t)}{dt} = \alpha_1 R(t) - \beta_1 X_1(t),$$

$$\frac{dX_i(t)}{dt} = \alpha_i X_{i-1}(t) - \beta_i X_i(t), \ i \geq 2,$$

where we assume that all the kinases are inactive at time $t = 0$, that is, we set $X_i(0) = 0$, $\forall i$. Following [83], we consider an exponentially decreasing input signal $R(t) = R(0) \exp(-\lambda t)$, $R(0) > 0$, for some parameter $\lambda > 0$, which is such that $\lambda \neq \beta_i$, $\forall i$.

- Use the method of variation of constants to deduce that

$$X_1(t) = \alpha_1 R(0) \frac{e^{-\lambda t} - e^{-\beta_1 t}}{\beta_1 - \lambda} \longrightarrow 0,$$

  exponentially fast as $t \to \infty$.

- Consider the density function f_i on $\mathbb{R}_+$,

$$f_i(t) = \frac{X_i(t)}{Z_i},$$

  where

$$Z_i = \int_0^\infty X_i(s)ds.$$

  Show that

$$Z_i = \frac{\alpha_i}{\beta_i} Z_{i-1}, \ i \geq 1.$$

- Deduce from this that

$$Z_i = \frac{R(0)}{\lambda} \prod_{k=1}^{i} \frac{\alpha_k}{\beta_k}.$$

- Use the definition of f_i to show that the signalling times τ_i satisfy the recursion

$$\tau_i = \tau_{i-1} + \frac{1}{\beta_i},$$

and deduce (4.7).

Chapter 5

Binding processes and transcription rates

Signaling pathways are instumental for gene transcription, through their action on transcription-controlling proteins, the so-called transcription factors (TF); see, e.g., [120]. TF interact with regulatory DNA motifs called promoter, enhancer or silencer sequences. Transcription is divided into three main phases: initiation, elongation and termination; we will present models describing the first phase. In eukaryotic cells, multiprotein complexes are formed; they are composed of RNA polymerase II and six general transcription factors. These TF are not gene specific and can thus be used for various genes. The activity of RNA polymerase, and of the general and gene-specific TF are controlled by signaling cascades, which are themselves activated by external stimuli. The DNA sequences of promoters and enhancers are composed of several distinct binding sites where gene specific transcription factors can bind, and thus enhance (positive regulation) or prevent (inhibition) transcription.

TF are themselves proteins encoded by genes which are under the control of other genes. The overall picture is given by a directed graph where the nodes are the genes, and where a directed arrow $A \to B$ from gene A to gene B indicates that A controls B. One can also indicate if this control is positive or negative. This intricate interaction graph is known as a **transcription network**. Actual knowledge of the human transcription network is very limited at the present time, but some well known transcription networks have been studied in detail in the biological literature; see, e.g., [4] for very interesting results.

This chapter aims at providing models of transcription rates, which are used as transition rates for Markov chains involving transcriptional steps. We explain how models from thermodynamics can help in understanding cooperativity and switching like behaviours.

5.1   Positive and negative control

Consider the toy model provided in section 1.2.2, where the expression of some gene B is modelled using the relation

$$\mathcal{M} \xrightarrow{\nu n} \emptyset, \quad \emptyset \xrightarrow{\mu} \mathcal{M},$$

where n denotes the number of proteins produced by the gene B. Let $E(t)$ be the mean number of B-proteins present in the cell at time t. We have seen in (1.10) that

$$\frac{\mathrm{d}E(t)}{\mathrm{d}t} = \mu - \nu E(t).$$

If B is under the control of A (see figure 5.1), it is meaningful to assume that the production rate μ is a function of the concentration v of A proteins. This is usually modelled using so-called **input functions** $f(v)$ such that

$$\mu = f(v).$$

If A is an **activator**, an increase of v leads to an increase of the production rate, so that f is increasing. On the other hand, if A is a **repressor**, f is decreasing. The most typical choices of input functions are the **Hill functions**; see, e.g., [4], which are defined by

$$f(v) = \frac{v^{\eta}}{K^{\eta} + v^{\eta}}, \tag{5.1}$$

when A is an activator. K is a positive constant and $\eta \in \mathbb{R}^{+}$ is the **Hill exponent**. When A is a repressor, the Hill function is

$$f(v) = \frac{K^{\eta}}{K^{\eta} + v^{\eta}}. \tag{5.2}$$

Usually, scientific papers use these functions without explaining the reasons for a particular choice. On the other hand, the literature also proposes thermodynamic models for such input functions; see, e.g., [101], [184], [181], [22], [92], [27], [20] or [19]. Section 5.12 provides tools from thermodynamics which shed light on these models, by explaining how functions like (5.1) or (5.2) can be obtained from binding processes. These functions are also used to model genetic switches where $f(v) \sim 0$ for $v < v_c$ and $f(v) \sim 1$ for $v > v_c$, for some critical threshold v_c. This can be achieved for large enough η; see, e.g., figure 1.7, or by using well designed biological processes (see section 7.2).

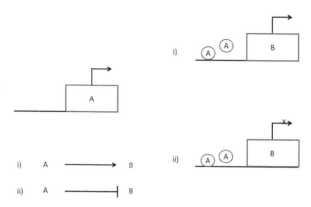

FIGURE 5.1: Gene A controls gene B. (i) When A is an activator, this control is positive, with, e.g., an input function given by (5.1), where v denotes the concentration of type A proteins. (ii) A is a repressor for B, with associated input function (5.2). These controls are realized by the binding of type A proteins on the B promoter.

5.2 Binding probabilities

We present basic models for processes involving the binding of ligand molecules on macromolecules, which are first level models for approaching the binding of TF to DNA. The possible binding sites may correspond to some regulatory region like a promoter. We follow essentially the monographs of [40] and [41], by presenting the material in a more statistically oriented language. We will also import some notions of statistical mechanics, statistics and neural network theory, and provide new results which shed light on the interplay between indexes of current practical use like the Hill coefficient and the cooperativity index. Let M be a macromolecule containing N binding sites $S = \{1, \cdots, N\}$ for a ligand. We will use the binary variables $n_i = 0, 1, i = 1, \cdots, N$ to describe the occupancy of the various sites: $n_i = 1$ means that site i is occupied by a ligand molecule, while $n_i = 0$ indicates that no molecule is bound at site i. The configuration space is denoted by $\Lambda = \{n = (n_i)_{1 \leq i \leq N}; \ n_i = 0, \ 1\}$, which has size $|\Lambda| = 2^N$.

We suppose in the sequel that a ligand molecule binds to some site i with a rate proportional to the **ligand concentration** v: we will hence consider

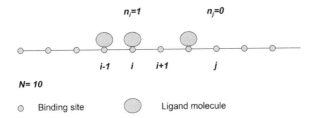

FIGURE 5.2: Graphical representation of a macromolecule containing N binding sites, where ligand molecules can bind. $n_i = 1$ means that site i is occupied by a ligand molecule, and $n_i = 0$ when it is free of ligand molecules. Such binding processes can model the binding of regulating proteins on a promoter; see figure 5.1.

probability distribution π of the form

$$\pi(n) = \frac{\mu(n)v^{|n|}}{Z(v)}, \quad n \in \Lambda, \tag{5.3}$$

for some weights $\mu(n) \geq 0$, $n \in \Lambda$, where $|n|$ denotes the number of bound sites in configuration n (also called the ligation number of configuration n), with

$$|n| = \sum_{i=1}^{N} n_i.$$

The normalization

$$Z(v) = \sum_{m \in \Lambda} \mu(m)v^{|m|}$$

is a polynomial in the variable v: the **binding polynomial** (see, e.g., [40] or [41]) is

$$\Psi(v) = \frac{Z(v)}{\mu(0)} = \sum_{k=0}^{N} v^k \Psi_k,$$

where

$$\Psi_k = \sum_{|n|=k} \frac{\mu(n)}{\mu(0)}. \tag{5.4}$$

As we have seen in the preceding chapters, chemical reactions are described mathematically using time-continuous Markov chains, and the related statistical equilibrium are described by the steady state distributions π. Most works in biochemistry proceed by establishing a free energy function H from first principles, and use Gibbs-Boltzmann distributions (see (2.17)) as steady states. We develop further these considerations in sections 5.3 and 6.

$\pi(n)$ gives the probability of seeing the system in configuration n at statistical equilibrium. The probability that $|n| = k$ is obtained by collecting all the configurations n such that $|n| = k$:

$$\pi(|n| = k) = \frac{v^k \sum_{|n|=k} \mu(n)}{Z(v)}.$$

The mathematical expectation of any function $f : \Lambda \longrightarrow \mathbb{R}$ is denoted by

$$\langle f \rangle_\pi = \sum_n f(n)\pi(n).$$

The following examples will play an important role in what follows. The mean of the occupation variable n_i is

$$\langle n_i \rangle_\pi = \sum_{n: \, n_i=1} \pi(n) = \pi(n_i = 1),$$

which is the probability that site i is occupied. When $i \neq j$, we will also use the second moments

$$\langle n_i n_j \rangle_\pi = \sum_{n: \, n_i=n_j=1} \pi(n) = \pi(n_i = n_j = 1)$$

and the covariances

$$\begin{aligned}
\mathrm{Cov}_\pi(n_i, n_j) &= \langle n_i n_j \rangle_\pi - \langle n_i \rangle_\pi \langle n_j \rangle_\pi \\
&= \pi(n_i = n_j = 1) - \pi(n_i = 1)\pi(n_j = 1).
\end{aligned}$$

The mean ligation number is obtained from the binding polynomial $\Psi(v)$ as

$$\begin{aligned}
\langle |n| \rangle_\pi &= \sum_n \pi(n)|n| = \sum_{k=0}^{N} k \sum_{n:|n|=k} \pi(n) \\
&= \sum_{k=1}^{N} k v^k \frac{\Psi_k}{\Psi(v)} = v\frac{\sum_{k=1}^{N} k v^{k-1} \Psi_k}{\Psi(v)} = v\frac{\frac{d\Psi(v)}{dv}}{\Psi(v)} \\
&= v\frac{d\ln(\Psi(v))}{dv}.
\end{aligned}$$

The **binding curve** is

$$N(v) = \langle |n| \rangle_\pi, \tag{5.5}$$

which is usually considered as a function of the log-concentration $\ln(v)$. A computation shows that

$$\frac{d\langle |n| \rangle_\pi}{d\ln(v)} = v\frac{d\langle |n| \rangle_\pi}{dv} = \mathrm{Var}_\pi(|n|), \tag{5.6}$$

so that $N(v)$ is always an **increasing function of** $\ln(v)$ and of v since $v > 0$.

The next notion of interest is the global **binding capacity** B, which is defined as the variance of the ligation number:

$$B = \text{Var}_\pi\left(\sum_{i=1}^N n_i\right) = \text{Var}_\pi(|n|) = \sum_{i=1}^N B_i,$$

where the site-specific binding capacities B_i are defined by

$$B_i = \text{Var}_\pi(n_i)(1 + \mathbb{E}_\pi(\bar{n}_i|n_i = 1) - \mathbb{E}_\pi(\bar{n}_i|n_i = 0));$$

see (5.8) below.

Conditional expectation

Let X and Y be discrete random variables taking values in $\mathbb{N}$. The conditional expectation of Y given that $\{X = n\}$ is defined by

$$\mathbb{E}(Y|X = n) = \sum_{k \in \mathbb{N}} kP(Y = k|X = n).$$

$\mathbb{E}(Y|X)$ will denote the related random variable, which is a function of X. The conditioning principle states that one can compute the expectation of the random variable Y as follows:

$$\begin{aligned}
\mathbb{E}(Y) &= \mathbb{E}(\mathbb{E}(Y|X)) \\
&= \sum_{n \in \mathbb{N}} \mathbb{E}(Y|X = n)P(X = n).
\end{aligned}$$

The variance of a sum of Bernoulli random variables

Let ε_j, $j = 1, \cdots, N$ be a collection of Bernoulli random variables. Set

$$\bar{\varepsilon}_i = \sum_{j \neq i} \varepsilon_j = \sum_{j=1}^{N} \varepsilon_j - \varepsilon_i.$$

Then

$$B = \mathrm{Var}(\sum_{i=1}^{N} \varepsilon_i) = \sum_{i=1}^{N} B_i,$$

where

$$B_i = \mathrm{Var}(\varepsilon_i) + \mathrm{Cov}(\varepsilon_i, \bar{\varepsilon}_i).$$

Furthermore,

$$\mathrm{Cov}(\varepsilon_i, \bar{\varepsilon}_i) = \mathrm{Var}(\varepsilon_i)(\mathbb{E}(\bar{\varepsilon}_i|\varepsilon_i = 1) - \mathbb{E}(\bar{\varepsilon}_i|\varepsilon_i = 0)), \tag{5.7}$$

so that

$$B_i = \mathrm{Var}(\varepsilon_i)(1 + \mathbb{E}(\bar{\varepsilon}_i|\varepsilon_i = 1) - \mathbb{E}(\bar{\varepsilon}_i|\varepsilon_i = 0)). \tag{5.8}$$

5.3 Gibbs-Boltzmann distributions

Let $H : \Lambda \longrightarrow \mathbb{R}$ be a free energy function which gives the binding energy $H(n)$ associated with n. We will explain in what follows how such energy functions model in some way the possible interactions between bound TF. When a system possesses such a free energy function, a standard assumption is that the probability of seeing the system in some state n is given by the Gibbs-Boltzmann distribution at inverse temperature β:

$$\pi_\beta(n) = \frac{\exp(-\beta H(n))v^{|n|}}{Z(\beta, v)}, \tag{5.9}$$

where $Z(\beta, v)$ is the **partition function** of the system,

$$Z(\beta, v) = \sum_{n \in \Lambda} \exp(-\beta H(n))v^{|n|}.$$

The reader can consult section 2.3.1 for more details on similar distributions.

Example 5.3.1 Suppose that all the configurations having a given ligation number k have the same free energy, that is, assume that $H(n)$ only depends on n through $|n|$, with $H(n) = V(|n|)$ for some function V. Then

$$\Psi(v) = \sum_{k=0}^{N} v^k \binom{N}{k} \exp(-\beta(V(k) - V(0))). \tag{5.10}$$

In this situation, the probability distribution of the random vector $(n_{\sigma(1)}, \cdots, n_{\sigma(N)})$, is independent of the permutation σ. The random variables are exchangeable.

Example 5.3.2 [Reference system] The reference system is defined as a system where the N occupation random variables n_i are i.i.d. Bernoulli; one can check that in this situation

$$H(n) = h \sum_{i=1}^{N} n_i,$$

for some constant h. Let $K = \exp(-\beta h)$. Then

$$\Psi(v) = \sum_{k=0}^{N} \binom{N}{k} v^k e^{-k\beta h} = (1 + Kv)^N,$$

and

$$
\begin{aligned}
\pi_\beta(n_1, \cdots, n_N) &= \frac{(vK)^{n_1} \cdots (vK)^{n_N}}{(1 + Kv)^N} \\
&= \frac{(vK)^{n_1}}{1 + Kv} \cdots \frac{(vK)^{n_N}}{1 + Kv}.
\end{aligned}
$$

The mean fraction of bound sites is

$$p = \frac{\langle |n| \rangle_{\pi_\beta}}{N} = \frac{Kv}{1 + Kv},$$

and the variance is such that

$$B_0(p) = \mathrm{Var}(\sum_{i=1}^{N} n_i) = Np(1 - p),$$

where the parameter of success of the Bernoulli random variables is p. Notice that the mean fraction of bound sites is independent of the number of binding sites.

Example 5.3.3 [Boltzmann machines] A basic model which describes interactions between binding sites is the Boltzmann machine model or the **Ising
model**

$$H(n) = -\sum_{i,j} J_{ij} n_i n_j - \sum_i h_i n_i, \qquad (5.11)$$

where the coefficients $J_{ij} = J_{ji}$ model pairwise interactions, and where the
parameters h_i are local field. This model is used in neural network theory,
due to its learning capacities; see, e.g., [1]. Usually, it is defined using a graph
of node set $S = \{1, \cdots, N\}$, and of edge set $\mathcal{E} = \{e = (i, j); J_{ij} \neq 0\}$. The
model is said to be ferro-magnetic when $J_{ij} \geq 0$. In this situation, assuming
that $h_i \equiv 0$ and $v > 1$, the most probable configuration is the fully occupied
one with $n_i \equiv 1$. Such models are of current use for modelling transcription
in prokaryotes; see, e.g., [27]. We will use such models when dealing with
regulation by λ phage repressors in section 5.13. One can extend this model
to a class containing many-body interactions, by setting

$$H(n) = -\sum_{S' \subset S} J_{S'} n_{S'}, \qquad (5.12)$$

where the occupation function $n_{S'}$ is defined for each subset S' of S by

$$n_{S'} = \prod_{i \in S'} n_i.$$

5.4 Site-specific Hill coefficients

It turns out that binding processes are usually **cooperative**: the binding
of a ligand molecule at some binding site i affects the binding of molecules at
other sites. Various notions of cooperativity exist; see, e.g., the discussion in
[96] and [97]. We focus mainly on cooperativity in the Hill sense, and introduce cooperativity in the microstate. The author of [40] introduces the Hill
coefficient at a given site i in chapters 3.1 and 3.2, using so-called *contracted
partition functions*, where some site is forced to be in a given ligation state. We
translate these notions here using conditional expectations of sums of binary
random variables; see formula (5.13) below.

Site-specific Hill coefficients

The Hill coefficient at site i is

$$\eta_{H,i}(v) = 1 + \mathbb{E}_\pi(\bar{n}_i | n_i = 1) - \mathbb{E}_\pi(\bar{n}_i | n_i = 0). \tag{5.13}$$

A direct interpretation of $\eta_{H,i}(v)$ is contained in (5.13): $\mathbb{E}_\pi(\bar{n}_i | n_i = 1) - \mathbb{E}_\pi(\bar{n}_i | n_i = 0)$ gives the gain in bound ligand molecules at sites different from i when adding a ligand molecule at site i. When this gain is positive (resp. negative), the system is said to exhibit positive (resp. negative) cooperativity at site i. We will come to these notions later. This can also be seen using the covariance as follows: set for convenience $Y = \bar{n}_i$ and $X = n_i$. The best affine prediction of Y by a random variable of the form $aX + b$ in the least square sense is obtained with

$$a^* = \frac{\mathrm{Cov}_\pi(X, Y)}{\mathrm{Var}_\pi(X)} = \mathbb{E}_\pi(\bar{n}_i | n_i = 1) - \mathbb{E}_\pi(\bar{n}_i | n_i = 0),$$

(see (5.7)), and

$$b^* = \mathbb{E}_\pi(Y) - a^* \mathbb{E}_\pi(X).$$

5.5   Cooperativity in the microstate*

Let i and j be two different binding sites. When the system is not cooperative, the occupation random variables n_i and n_j should be independent or decorrelated, with $\mathrm{Cov}_\pi(n_i, n_j) = 0$, or, equivalently, with $\langle n_i n_j \rangle_\pi = \langle n_i \rangle_\pi \langle n_j \rangle_\pi$. When the binding process exhibits some kind of positive cooperativity, one might be tempted to say that there exists a pair of binding sites (i, j) such that the probability that both sites are occupied $\pi(n_i = n_j = 1) = \langle n_i n_j \rangle_\pi$ is larger than the product of the individual occupation probabilities $\pi(n_i = 1)\pi(n_j = 1) = \langle n_i \rangle_\pi \langle n_j \rangle_\pi$ (see, e.g., [41]), that is, one should have

$$\mathrm{Cov}_\pi(n_i, n_j) \geq 0,$$

with a strict inequality for at least some pair of binding sites. Likewise, negative cooperativity between the occupation variables at sites i and j should occur when

$$\pi(n_i = n_j = 1) \leq \pi(n_i = 1)\pi(n_j = 1).$$

In statistics, one says that the random variables n_i are positively and negatively correlated. Formulas (5.8) and (5.13) show that

$$\text{Cov}_\pi(n_i, n_j) \geq 0, \; j \neq i \;\; \Rightarrow \;\; \eta_{H,i} \geq 1. \tag{5.14}$$

Hence, when the occupation random variables n_i and n_j are positively correlated for $j \neq i$, one has positive cooperativity in the Hill sense at site i. It turns out that statistical mechanics provides criteria ensuring that a given system exhibits cooperativity.

Example 5.5.1 Consider a ferromagnetic Boltzmann machine or Ising model with positive coupling coefficients; see (5.12). A function $f(n)$ is said to be increasing when $f(n) \leq f(n')$ for all configurations n and n' such that $n_i \leq n'_i$, $i \in S$. For ferro-magnetic systems, the **Fortuin-Kastelyn-Ginibre** (FKG) inequality states that

$$\langle fg \rangle_{\pi_\beta} \geq \langle f \rangle_{\pi_\beta} \langle g \rangle_{\pi_\beta},$$

for all pairs of increasing functions f and g; see, e.g., [56] and [77]. Let $S' \subset S$, and consider the occupation variable $n_{S'} = \prod_{i \in S'} n_i$, which is a typical example of an increasing function. In particular, when $S' = \{i, j\}$, with $i \neq j$, the FKG inequality shows that the binding process is cooperative since $\langle n_i n_j \rangle_{\pi_\beta} = \pi_\beta(n_i = n_j = 1)$ and $\langle n_i \rangle_{\pi_\beta} = \pi_\beta(n_i = 1)$. Moreover, let A and B be two disjoint subsets of S, with $n_{A \cup B} = n_A n_B$. The FKG inequality yields furthermore that

$$\pi_\beta(n_A = n_B = 1) \geq \pi_\beta(n_A = 1)\pi_\beta(n_B = 1),$$

or, in words,

$$\text{Prob}(A \text{ and } B \text{ are simultaneously occupied})$$

$$\geq \text{Prob}(A \text{ is occupied}) \, \text{Prob}(B \text{ is occupied}).$$

5.6 The sigmoidal nature of the binding curve*

Recall that the binding curve (5.5) is the plot of $N(v)$ versus $\ln(v)$. In most experiments, it turns out that this curve has an S-shape, that is, is non-decreasing with an inflexion point v_c such that

$$\frac{d^2 N(v)}{d\ln(v)^2} \geq 0, \;\; v \leq v_c,$$

and

$$\frac{\mathrm{d}^2 N(v)}{\mathrm{d}\ln(v)^2} \leq 0, \quad v \geq v_c.$$

The reader can consult [97] and [96] where many interesting results concerning the shape of binding curves are provided. These results deal mostly with properties of binding polynomial coefficients, which are, however, difficult to handle mathematically. We will check the S-shape within the family of ferromagnetic Boltzmann machines models (see (5.11) and example 5.5.1) and also provide examples from systems biology in sections 5.13 and 6.1. A computation shows that

$$
\begin{aligned}
\frac{\mathrm{d}^2 N(v)}{\mathrm{d}\ln(v)^2} &= \langle |n|^3 \rangle_\pi - 3\langle |n|^2 \rangle_\pi \langle |n| \rangle_\pi + 2\langle |n| \rangle_\pi^3 \\
&= \langle (|n| - \langle |n| \rangle_\pi)^3 \rangle_\pi.
\end{aligned}
$$

When π is a Gibbs-Boltzmann distribution, this last function is known as an Ursell function of order three; see, e.g., [111]. It is difficult to work out the above expression. For Boltzmann machines, it turns out that statistical mechanics provides useful moment inequalities which can help in our setting. Recall that the free energy function associated with a Boltzmann machine is

$$H(n) = -\sum_{i \neq j} J_{ij} n_i n_i - \sum_i h_i n_i.$$

The related Gibbs measure

$$\pi_\beta(n) = \frac{e^{-\beta H(n)} v^{|n|}}{Z(\beta, v)},$$

can be defined using the modified free-energy function

$$
\begin{aligned}
\bar{H}(n) &= H(n) - \sum_i \frac{\ln(v)}{\beta} n_i \\
&= -\sum_{i \neq j} J_{ij} n_i n_j - \sum_i \bar{h}_i n_i,
\end{aligned}
$$

where we set

$$\bar{h}_i = h_i + \frac{\ln(v)}{\beta}.$$

The Gibbs measure then becomes

$$\pi_\beta(n) = \frac{e^{-\beta \bar{H}(n)}}{Z(\beta, v)}.$$

Let $\hat{h}_i = \sum_{j \neq i} J_{ij}$. For ferromagnetic Boltzmann machines, the so-called **Griffiths-Hurst-Sherman** (GHS) inequality states that for arbitrary sites i, j and k,

$$\langle(n_i - \langle n_i \rangle_{\pi_\beta})((n_j - \langle n_j \rangle_{\pi_\beta})(n_k - \langle n_k \rangle_{\pi_\beta}))\rangle_{\pi_\beta} \geq 0,$$

when $\hat{h}_i + \bar{h}_i \leq 0$, $\forall i$, with the reverse inequality in the opposite case; see, e.g., [45]. The GHS inequality and the identity

$$
\begin{aligned}
\langle(|n| - \langle |n| \rangle_{\pi_\beta})^3\rangle_{\pi_\beta} &= \langle(\sum_i (n_i - \langle n_i \rangle_{\pi_\beta}))^3\rangle_{\pi_\beta} \\
&= \sum_{ijk} \langle(n_i - \langle n_i \rangle_{\pi_\beta})((n_j - \langle n_j \rangle_{\pi_\beta})(n_k - \langle n_k \rangle_{\pi_\beta}))\rangle_{\pi_\beta}
\end{aligned}
$$

lead to the inequality

$$\langle(|n| - \langle |n| \rangle_{\pi_\beta})^3\rangle_{\pi_\beta} \geq 0,$$

when $\hat{h}_i + \bar{h}_i \leq 0$, $\forall i$. The proof of this famous inequality is tricky (see [111]) and its extension to other models is not obvious mathematically. Hence, when $\hat{h}_i + h_i \equiv h_0$, one obtains that the binding curve associated with a ferromagnetic Boltzmann machine has an S-shape, of inflexion point given by

$$v_c = \exp(-\beta h_0).$$

5.7   Cooperativity in the Hill sense

The third quantity of interest besides $\langle |n| \rangle_\pi$ and $B = \mathrm{Var}_\pi(|n|)$ is the **affinity function** $^v K$,

$$^v K = \frac{\langle |n| \rangle_\pi}{v(N - \langle |n| \rangle_\pi)}, \tag{5.15}$$

which corresponds to the following ratios of concentrations:

$$^v K = \frac{[\text{sites bound by a ligand molecule}]}{[\text{sites free of ligand molecules}][\text{ligand molecules}]}.$$

With this interpretation, $^v K$ is the equilibrium constant of the reaction

$$\text{site free} + \text{ligand} \longleftrightarrow \text{site bound};$$

see, e.g., [40] for more details. The **affinity plot** is the logarithm of $^v K$ versus the logarithm of the ligand activity $\ln(v)$. In the reference system, where all the occupation random variables are i.i.d. Bernoulli of success parameter $p = vK/(1 + vK)$, one obtains that

$$^vK = K,$$

showing that the affinity function is constant.

The **Hill plot** is the logarithm of the ratio $\langle |n| \rangle_\pi / (N - \langle |n| \rangle_\pi)$ versus the logarithm of the ligand activity. When the random variables n_i, $i = 1, \cdots, N$ are i.i.d., the associated Hill plot is a straight line of unit slope. Notice that

$$\ln\left(\frac{\langle |n| \rangle_\pi}{N - \langle |n| \rangle_\pi}\right) = \ln(^vK) + \ln(v).$$

The **Hill coefficient of cooperativity** $\eta_H(v)$ is the slope of the Hill plot, that is,

$$\eta_H(v) = \frac{d \ln\left(\frac{\langle |n| \rangle_\pi}{N - \langle |n| \rangle_\pi}\right)}{d \ln(v)} = 1 + \frac{d \ln(^vK)}{d \ln(v)}. \tag{5.16}$$

The Hill coefficient should be considered as a **function of the log-concentration** $\ln(v)$, and was defined by Hill [84] to study double logarithmic plots related to oxygen and hemoglobin binding curves. The Hill coefficient is directly related to the binding capacity: a computation shows that

$$\eta_H(v) = \frac{NB}{\langle |n| \rangle_\pi (N - \langle |n| \rangle_\pi)} = \frac{B}{N\bar{p}(1 - \bar{p})}, \tag{5.17}$$

where

$$\bar{p} = \frac{1}{N} \langle |n| \rangle_\pi = \frac{1}{N} \sum_{i=1}^{N} \pi(n_i = 1).$$

$\eta_H(v)$ is such that

$$0 \leq \eta_H(v) \leq N, \tag{5.18}$$

for positive $v > 0$. The upper bound follows from (5.17) since

$$\begin{aligned}
\eta_H(v) &= N\frac{\langle |n|^2 \rangle_\pi - (\langle |n| \rangle_\pi)^2}{\langle |n| \rangle_\pi (N - \langle |n| \rangle_\pi)} \\
&\leq N\frac{N\langle |n| \rangle_\pi - (\langle |n| \rangle_\pi)^2}{\langle |n| \rangle_\pi (N - \langle |n| \rangle_\pi)} = N,
\end{aligned}$$

where we use the fact that $|n| \leq N$ for N binding sites.

Cooperativity in the Hill sense

- When $\eta_H(v) > 1$ for all $v > 0$, we have positive cooperativity in the sense of Hill.

- Likewise, when $\eta_H(v) < 1$ for all $v > 0$, we have negative cooperativity.

- The special case where $\eta_H(v) \equiv 1$ is synonomous with non-cooperativity.

Hill [84] proposed $\eta_H(v)$ as an indicator of cooperativity: let $N(v)$ be a binding curve (see (5.5)) which should contain information about the cooperative behaviour of some system. Hill proposed comparing $N(v)$ to Hill functions (5.1), by setting

$$N(v) = \langle |n| \rangle_\pi = \frac{v^\eta}{K^\eta + v^\eta} N, \tag{5.19}$$

for positive parameters K and η. Hence,

$$\ln\left(\frac{N(v)}{N - N(v)}\right) = \eta \ln(v) - \eta \ln(K),$$

which explains the idea which is behind the definition (5.16). Equation (5.19) compares the binding probability π to a probability μ for which

$$\mu(|n| = N) = \frac{v^\eta}{K^\eta + v^\eta}, \ \ \mu(|n| = 0) = \frac{K^\eta}{K^\eta + v^\eta},$$

and

$$\mu(|n| = k) = 0, \ \ \forall 0 < k < N,$$

so that

$$\langle |n| \rangle_\mu = \frac{v^\eta}{K^\eta + v^\eta} N.$$

One understands intuitively why this last probability distribution exhibits a high cooperative behaviour: the intermediate configurations with $|n| \neq 0, N$ have zero probability, leading to **all or none states**. The related Hill coefficient associated with μ is

$$\eta_H(v) = \eta.$$

This shows that the Hill coefficient $\eta_H(v)$ associated with a probability measure π provides a meaningful cooperativity index when the intermediate ligation states have effectively low probabilities. This also shows that one should use this index with great care if this is not the case. In practice, scientists use $\eta_H(\bar{v})$ where the intermediate concentration $\bar{v}$ is associated with a mean ligation number which is halfway between the minimum and the maximum ligation states; see, e.g., [10].

The Hill coefficient is not only used for measuring cooperativity in binding processes. One can use it for **dose-responses curves** $V(v)$, $v > 0$, where $0 \leq V(v)/V(\infty) \leq 1$ can often be seen as a probability distribution function; see, e.g, [96], [97] or [76]. In this general situation, the Hill coefficient is, when V is differentiable,

$$\eta_H(v) = \frac{d \ln(\frac{V(v)}{V(\infty)-V(v)})}{d \ln(v)}. \tag{5.20}$$

Notice that for binding process, $N(\infty) \neq N$ in general, so that these two notions do not necessarily coincide. Section 8 considers such Hill coefficients to study the steepness of signalling switches.

5.8 $\eta_H(v)$ as an indicator of cooperativity

Recall that

$$\eta_H(v) = \frac{B}{B_0(\bar{p})} = \frac{\text{Var}_\pi(\sum n_i)}{N\bar{p}(1 - \bar{p})},$$

with

$$\text{Var}_\pi\left(\sum n_i\right) = \sum_i \text{Var}_\pi(n_i) + \sum_{i \neq j} \text{Cov}_\pi(n_i, n_j).$$

Positive cooperativity in the microstate holds when

$$\text{Cov}_\pi(n_i, n_j) \geq 0, \tag{5.21}$$

when $i \neq j$, with a strict inequality for at least a pair of sites; see section 5.5. We thus can suspect that $\eta_H(v)$ can be large when (5.21) is satisfied. However, (5.21) is not sufficient to ensure positive cooperativity in the sense of Hill: let $p_i = \langle n_i \rangle_\pi$. Then, since

$$\frac{\sum_i p_i^2}{N} > \left(\frac{\sum_i p_i}{N}\right)^2,$$

for non-constant $p = (p_i)$, one deduces that

$$N \sum_i p_i(1 - p_i) < \left(\sum_i p_i\right)\left(N - \sum_i p_i\right).$$

The statement follows from the above inequality since

$$\eta_H(v) = \frac{N \sum_i p_i(1 - p_i) + N \sum_{i \neq j} \text{Cov}_\pi(n_i, n_j)}{\left(\sum_i p_i\right)\left(N - \sum_i p_i\right)}.$$

On the other hand, if $p_i = p$, $\forall i$, for some constant p, as it is the case for exchangeable occupation variables (see example 5.3.1) one has positive cooperativity in the Hill sense when (5.21) holds for any pair $i \neq j$.

5.9 The cooperativity index

The authors of [109] and [70] proposed an index which can be used to check cooperativity (see, e.g., [96] and [97]), or to check the steepness of dose-response curves $V(v)$, $v > 0$; see [76]). Chapters 7 and 8 study switches where dose-responses curves switch abruptly from a low saturation level to a high saturation level in the vicinity of some critical concentration v_c. The so-called cooperativity index provides a measure of the steepness of $V(v)$. When $V(v)/V(\infty)$ can be seen as a probability distribution function of $v > 0$, one can look, for given $\frac{1}{2} < p < 1$, at the related quantiles $v_{1-p} \leq v_p$ defined by $p = V(v_p)/V(\infty)$ and $1 - p = V(v_{1-p})/V(\infty)$. The **cooperativity index**, which is also called the **Koshland cooperativity measure** I (see [96]) is obtained when $p = 0.9$ and is

$$I = \frac{\ln(81)}{\ln\left(\frac{v_{0.9}}{v_{0.1}}\right)}. \tag{5.22}$$

More generally, one might define the index

$$I_p = \frac{2\ln\left(\frac{p}{1-p}\right)}{\ln\left(\frac{v_p}{v_{1-p}}\right)}.$$

When $p = 0.9$, $\ln(v_p/v_{1-p})$ provides a measure of the dose difference one must consider to move $V(v)/V(\infty)$ from a low 10% saturation level to a high 90% saturation level. The curve is **steep when I_p is large**, that is, when v_p/v_{1-p} is close to 1. Notice that this index has some drawbacks: for example, if one shifts the curve $V(v)$ by an amount $\triangle > 0$, the ratio moves from v_p/v_{1-p} to $(v_p + \triangle)/(v_{1-p} + \triangle)$, which is decreasing as a function of $\triangle$; see, e.g., [76] for a very instructive discussion.

When $V(v)/V(\infty)$ is a Hill function, that is, when

$$\frac{V(v)}{V(\infty)} = \frac{v^\eta}{K^\eta + v^\eta},$$

a direct computation shows that

$$\eta = I_p, \ \forall p > \frac{1}{2}.$$

The cooperativity index thus recovers the Hill exponent when the dose-response curve is a Hill function. The following computation establishes a link between η_H and I_p. First notice that I_p is

$$I_p = \frac{\ln(p) - \ln(1-p)}{\ln(v_p) - \ln(v_{1-p})} - \frac{\ln(1-p) - \ln(p)}{\ln(v_p) - \ln(v_{1-p})},$$

which can be rewritten as

$$I_p = \frac{\ln(V(v_p)) - \ln(V(v_{1-p}))}{\ln(v_p) - \ln(v_{1-p})} - \frac{\ln(V(\infty) - V(v_p)) - \ln(V(\infty) - V(v_{1-p}))}{\ln(v_p) - \ln(v_{1-p})}.$$

Hence

$$
\begin{aligned}
I_p &= \frac{1}{\ln(v_p) - \ln(v_{1-p})} \int_{v_{1-p}}^{v_p} \frac{d\ln\left(\frac{V(v)}{V(\infty) - V(v)}\right)}{dv} dv \\
&= \frac{1}{\ln(v_p) - \ln(v_{1-p})} \int_{v_{1-p}}^{v_p} v \frac{d\ln\left(\frac{V(v)}{V(\infty) - V(v)}\right)}{dv} \frac{dv}{v} \\
&= \frac{1}{\ln(v_p) - \ln(v_{1-p})} \int_{v_{1-p}}^{v_p} \eta_H(v) \frac{dv}{v} \\
&\leq \sup_{v>0} \eta_H(v) \frac{\int_{v_{1-p}}^{v_p} \frac{dv}{v}}{\ln(v_p) - \ln(v_{1-p})} = \sup_{v>0} \eta_H(v),
\end{aligned}
$$

which yields the upper bound

$$I_p \leq \sup_{v>0} \eta_H(v). \tag{5.23}$$

The above inequality shows that ultrasensitivity with high values of I_p implies positive cooperativity in the Hill sense. Let $\bar{\eta}_H$ be the Hill coefficient expressed as a function of $\ln(v)$, that is, set $\eta_H(v) = \bar{\eta}_H(\ln(v))$. Then

$$
\begin{aligned}
I_p &= \frac{1}{\ln(v_p) - \ln(v_{1-p})} \int_{v_{1-p}}^{v_p} \eta_H(v) \frac{dv}{v} \\
&= \frac{1}{\ln(v_p) - \ln(v_{1-p})} \int_{v_{1-p}}^{v_p} \bar{\eta}_H(\ln(v)) \frac{dv}{v} \\
&= \frac{1}{\ln(v_p) - \ln(v_{1-p})} \int_{\ln(v_{1-p})}^{\ln(v_p)} \bar{\eta}_H(y) dy,
\end{aligned}
$$

is the average of the Hill coefficient $\bar{\eta}_H$ between $\ln(v_{1-p})$ and $\ln(v_p)$.

5.10 Macroscopic cooperativity

When $\pi = \pi_\beta$ for some free energy function H, the binding process can also be studied macroscopically, by forgetting in some sense the binding of ligand molecules at specific sites. The usual approach consists in defining an effective binding free energy $\triangle G_k$ as follows:

$$\binom{N}{k} \exp(-\beta \triangle G_k) = \Psi_k = \sum_{|n|=k} \exp(-\beta(H(n) - H(0))). \qquad (5.24)$$

Let us introduce the **stepwise binding constants**

$$\kappa_k = \frac{\Psi_k}{\binom{N}{k}} \frac{\binom{N}{k-1}}{\Psi_{k-1}} = \exp(-\beta(\triangle G_k - \triangle G_{k-1})),$$

with

$$\Psi_k = \binom{N}{k} \kappa_1 \cdots \kappa_k,$$

where Ψ_k has been defined in (5.4). Cooperative systems are also characterized as systems where the constants κ_k change with the ligation number k: for example, if the sequence (κ_k) is increasing (resp. decreasing), one speaks sometimes of positive (resp. negative) cooperativity; see, e.g., [40]. The authors of [96] and [97] provided detailed comparisons of various notions of cooperativity using similar affinity constants. One might be tempted to be more pragmatic by considering only criteria leading to practical ways of checking if a system exhibits some kind of cooperativity. Practically, the literature often ignores the intermediate values κ_k, $k = 2, \cdots, N-1$ to focus on κ_1 and κ_N: in this case, one has positive cooperativity when $\kappa_N > \kappa_1$ and negative cooperativity when $\kappa_N < \kappa_1$.

Exercise 5.10.1 This material is taken from [40]. Consider a macromolecule containing two binding sites, and assume that the binding process is described by a Gibbs-Boltzmann distribution. The binding polynomial is

$$\Psi(v) = 1 + \Psi_1 v + \Psi_2 v^2.$$

Set

$$K_1 = \exp(-\beta(H(1,0) - H(0,0))) \text{ and } K_2 = \exp(-\beta(H(0,1) - H(0,0))),$$

where $H(n) = H(n_1, n_2)$ is the binding free energy function. Let c_{12} be the interaction constant defined by

$$\Psi_2 = c_{12}K_1K_2.$$

Let κ_1 and κ_2 be the stepwise global binding constants.

- Check that
$$\kappa_1 = \frac{\Psi_1}{2} \text{ and } \kappa_2 = \frac{2\Psi_2}{\Psi_1}.$$

- Establish the formulas
$$\langle|n|\rangle_{\pi_\beta} = \frac{\Psi_1 v + 2\Psi_2 v^2}{\Psi(v)}, \quad B = \frac{\Psi_1 v + 4\Psi_2 v^2 + \Psi_1\Psi_2 v^3}{\Psi(v)^2},$$

$$^v K = \frac{\Psi_1 + 2\Psi_2 v}{2 + \Psi_1 v}, \quad \eta_H(v) = 1 + \frac{\kappa_2 v}{1 + \kappa_2 v} - \frac{\kappa_1 v}{1 + \kappa_1 v},$$

$$\pi_\beta(n_1 = 1) = \frac{K_1 v (1 + c_{12}K_2 v)}{1 + (K_1 + K_2)v + c_{12}K_1 K_2 v^2}.$$

- Show that the site-specific Hill coefficient at site $i = 1$ is

$$\eta_{H,1} = \frac{d\ln\left(\frac{\pi_\beta(n_1=1)}{\pi_\beta(n_1=0)}\right)}{d\ln(v)}.$$

- Show that
$$\text{Cov}_{\pi_\beta}(n_1, n_2) > 0 \text{ if and only if } c_{12} > 1.$$

- The macroscopic condition of positive cooperativity requires that $\kappa_2 > \kappa_1$. Show that it is equivalent to the condition

$$4c_{12}K_1K_2 > (K_1 + K_2)^2.$$

- Deduce that these two notions of positive cooperativity are not equivalent.

5.11   The case $N = 3^*$

We present here some exact formulas for three binding sites, borrowing some material of [40]: the binding polynomial is of the form

$$\Psi(v) = 1 + \Psi_1 v + \Psi_2 v^2 + \Psi_3 v^3.$$

Introduce the constants

$$
\begin{aligned}
K_1 &= \exp(-\beta(H(1,0,0) - H(0,0,0))), \\
K_2 &= \exp(-\beta(H(0,1,0) - H(0,0,0))), \\
K_3 &= \exp(-\beta(H(0,0,1) - H(0,0,0))),
\end{aligned}
$$

where, for example, $n = (1,0,0)$ is the configuration such that $n_1 = 1$, $n_2 = 0$ and $n_3 = 0$. Introduce interaction constants c_{ij} between sites i and j as follows:

$$
\begin{aligned}
\Psi_1 &= K_1 + K_2 + K_3, \\
\Psi_2 &= c_{12}K_1K_2 + c_{13}K_1K_3 + c_{23}K_2K_3, \\
\Psi_3 &= c_{123}K_1K_2K_3,
\end{aligned}
$$

where c_{123} is the interaction constant associated with the fully occupied configuration. Then

$$
\langle |n| \rangle_{\pi_\beta} = \frac{\Psi_1 v + 2\Psi_2 v^2 + 3\Psi_3 v^3}{1 + \Psi_1 v + \Psi_2 v^2 + \Psi_3 v^3},
$$

$$
B = \frac{\Psi_1 v + 4\Psi_2 v^2 + (\Psi_1\Psi_2 + 9\Psi_3)v^3 + 4\Psi_1\Psi_3 v^4 + \Psi_2\Psi_3 v^5}{(1 + \Psi_1 v + \Psi_2 v^2 + \Psi_3 v^3)^2},
$$

and

$$
{}^v K = \frac{\Psi_1 + 2\Psi_2 v + 3\Psi_3 v^2}{3 + 2\Psi_1 v + \Psi_2 v^2}.
$$

Note that

$$
{}^v K = \kappa_1 \frac{1 + 2\kappa_2 v + \kappa_2\kappa_3 v^2}{1 + 2\kappa_1 v + \kappa_1\kappa_2 v^2},
$$

where the κ_i are the previously introduced stepwise binding constants. The Hill coefficient is

$$
\eta_H(v) = 1 + \frac{2\kappa_2 v(1 + \kappa_3 v)}{1 + 2\kappa_2 v + \kappa_2\kappa_3 v^2} - \frac{2\kappa_1 v(1 + \kappa_2 v)}{1 + 2\kappa_1 v + \kappa_1\kappa_2 v^2}.
$$

One can define site specific affinity functions:

$$
\begin{aligned}
{}^v K_1 &= K_1 \frac{1 + (c_{12}K_2 + c_{13}K_3)v + c_{123}K_2K_3 v^2}{1 + (K_2 + K_3)v + c_{23}K_2K_3 v^2} \\
{}^v K_2 &= K_2 \frac{1 + (c_{12}K_1 + c_{23}K_3)v + c_{123}K_1K_3 v^2}{1 + (K_1 + K_3)v + c_{13}K_1K_3 v^2} \\
{}^v K_3 &= K_3 \frac{1 + (c_{13}K_1 + c_{23}K_2)v + c_{123}K_1K_2 v^2}{1 + (K_1 + K_2)v + c_{12}K_1K_2 v^2}.
\end{aligned}
$$

The site specific binding probabilities are given by the formula

$$
\pi_\beta(n_i = 1) = \frac{{}^v K_i v}{1 + {}^v K_i v}.
$$

The Hill coefficient at site i can be computed as

$$\eta_{H,i}(v) = 1 + \frac{d\ln(^v K_i)}{d\ln(v)}. \tag{5.25}$$

These mathematical expressions will be useful in section 5.13.

Exercise 5.11.1 A macromolecule contains N binding sites for a ligand X. Let $v > 0$ be the ligand concentration, and let n_i, $i = 1, \cdots, N$ be the related occupation random variables. Let π be a probability defined on the binding configurations $n = (n_1, \cdots, n_N)$, of the form

$$\pi(n) = \frac{\mu(n)v^{|n|}}{Z(v)},$$

where $|n| = \sum_i n_i$. Let

$$N(v) = \langle |n| \rangle_\pi = \sum_n |n|\pi(n),$$

be the function giving the mean ligation number. Prove the following assertions:

-
$$\frac{dN(v)}{d\ln(v)} = \mathrm{Var}_\pi(|n|),$$

  where $\mathrm{Var}_\pi(|n|)$ is the variance of the ligation number.

-
$$\begin{aligned}
\frac{d^2 N(v)}{d\ln(v)^2} &= \langle |n|^3 \rangle_\pi - 3\langle |n|^2 \rangle_\pi \langle |n| \rangle_\pi + 2\langle |n| \rangle_\pi^3 \\
&= \langle (|n| - \langle |n| \rangle_\pi)^3 \rangle_\pi.
\end{aligned}$$

- The Hill plot is a straight line when the occupation random variables are i.i.d.

- The Hill coefficient $\eta_H(v)$ is related to the ligation number variance as

$$\eta_H(v) = \frac{\mathrm{Var}_\pi(|n|)}{N\bar{p}(1-\bar{p})},$$

  where $\bar{p} = \langle |n| \rangle_\pi / N$.

Exercise 5.11.2 We adopt the framework of example 5.11.1. Let π be a probability measure on the configuration space such that

$$\pi(|n| = k) = 0, \text{ for } 0 < k < N,$$

$$\pi(|n| = 0) = \frac{K^\eta}{K^\eta + v^\eta} \text{ and } \pi(|n| = N) = \frac{v^\eta}{K^\eta + v^\eta},$$

for positive parameters η and K, which assigns positive probabilities only to the empty and fully occupied configurations. Show that the Hill coefficient and the cooperativity index are such that

$$\eta_H(v) \equiv \eta \text{ and } I_p \equiv \eta.$$

5.12 Transcription rates for basic models

We consider here a simple model of transcription which assumes that ligand molecules can bind stochastically to a macromolecule containing N binding sites. This kind of model can be applied to model transcription in prokaryotes, where the binding sites are associated with some operator. When the ligand molecules enhance transcription, the operator's occupation determines the level of transcription. We will provide specific biological examples later. The reader can consult, e.g., [27], where more involved models of transcription in prokaryotes are presented, which make strong use of models from Boltzmann machines theory. Transcription in eukaryotes involves the binding of TF to specific DNA sequences, but is more complex, see, e.g., [11], [134] or [22]. We will provide precise biological examples in this setting.

In most applications, the **transcription rate** $T(v)$, that is, the rate at which mRNAs are produced, is modelled using the average ligation number

$$T(v) = \frac{\langle |n| \rangle_\pi}{N},$$

where v denotes the ligand concentration, with

$$\frac{\langle |n| \rangle_\pi}{N} = \frac{\sum_{i=1}^{N} \pi(n_i = 1)}{N} = \frac{v d \ln(\Psi(v))}{N dv},$$

where $\Psi(v)$ is the binding polynomial.

Transcription is initiated when the promoter is ON. In prokaryotes, the promoter is active when the operator occupation is in a given set of states $\Lambda_1 \subset \Lambda = \{(n_1, \cdots, n_N); \ n_i = 0, \ 1\}$. In this case, the transcription rate is often modelled as the probability

$$T(v) = \pi(n \in \Lambda_1);$$

see, e.g., [27], [92] or section 5.13. For example, some models propose transcription rates of the form

$$T(v) = \pi(|n| > k_0),$$

for some threshold k_0, so that the gene is active when the number of bound regulatory proteins is larger than k_0.

Positive and negative regulation

Assume that some gene A controls a gene B, as discussed in section 5.1. Recall that one starts from the reaction

$$\mathcal{M} \xrightarrow{\nu n} \emptyset, \quad \emptyset \xrightarrow{\mu} \mathcal{M},$$

so that the mean number of B-proteins $E(t)$ solves the o.d.e.

$$\frac{\mathrm{d}E(t)}{\mathrm{d}t} = f(v) - \nu E(t),$$

for some input function f, with $\mu = f(v)$.

For positive regulation, a natural input function is

$$f(v) = \frac{\langle |n| \rangle_\pi}{N},$$

which means that the transcriptional activity is directly related to the mean promoter's occupancy. Likewise, one can choose

$$f(v) = 1 - \frac{\langle |n| \rangle_\pi}{N}$$

when the control of A on B is negative.

When $A = B$, the gene is **auto-regulated**, and positive regulation leads to a so-called **positive feedback loop**, while negative regulation leads to a **negative feedback loop**. Negative regulation can accelerate convergence to steady state, and can provide robustness with respect to perturbations;

see, e.g., [30] and [4] where these notions are considered using deterministic models. Genetic networks can contain negative feedback loops to prevent large stochastic fluctuations; see, e.g., [12] or [152], [113] or section 3.5 for an illustration in a simple case. We will consider stochastic systems and check the effect of negative feedback loops on noise propagation in section 12.5. On the other hand, positive feedback loops are thought to slow convergence and provide bistability or even multistationarity; see, e.g., [92], [11] or [161]. Both modes can be used to build genetic switches; see, e.g., [81] or section 5.13. Positive and negative regulation can also lead to shifts in noise frequencies: the authors of [159] showed how negative regulation shifts the noise to higher frequencies, allowing better noise filtering by gene networks. The reader can consult [8], where the effect of network structures on noise frequencies is considered both theoretically and empirically. The global picture is, however, not so clear: the authors of [30] and [71] provide interesting examples where negative feedback loops can induce instabilities, and also examples where positive feedback loops can contribute to the stability of gene networks.

In the above setting, the promoter is always active, with a production rate $f(v)$ depending on the concentration of A-proteins. If the gene is self-regulated, as described by the relation

$$\mathcal{M} \xrightarrow{\nu x} \emptyset, \quad \emptyset \xrightarrow{\mu_l} \mathcal{M}, \quad l \in \{0,1\}, \quad \mathcal{O}_0 + \mathcal{M} \underset{\kappa(x)}{\overset{g(x)}{\rightleftarrows}} \mathcal{O}_1, \tag{5.26}$$

where x denotes the number of proteins (see chapter 1), the promoter switches randomly between the OFF and ON phases. Positive auto-regulation can be modelled by

$$g(x) = \frac{\langle |n| \rangle_\pi}{N} \quad \text{and} \quad \kappa(x) \equiv \kappa_0,$$

for some constant κ_0, for $v = x$. Likewise, negative regulation is obtained by setting

$$\kappa(x) = \frac{\langle |n| \rangle_\pi}{N} \quad \text{and} \quad g(x) \equiv g_0.$$

Notice that we might also model negative (resp. positive) regulation by choosing g to be decreasing (resp. increasing) with constant κ.

5.13   A genetic switch: regulation by λ phage repressor

Phage lambda is a virus (bacteria eater), which infects the bacterium *E. coli* by injecting its DNA, which is then integrated into the bacterium genome; see figure 5.3. We present here a mathematical model developed in [2] and [156] describing the genetic switch between the phage lambda *lytic* and *lysogenic* phenotypes, which are characterised by the expression levels of the *cro* and *cI* genes. In prokaryotes, genes are switched ON and OFF by regulatory proteins which interact with specific DNA sequences at operator sites; the state of the system then oscillates randomly between the two phenotypes.

In the lysogenic mode, the *cI* gene is synthesised, and the produced repressor proteins occupy the two O_{R1} and O_{R2} operators, leading to the repression of the *cro* gene (see figure 5.4). The phage can switch into the lytic mode, where the repressors are destroyed. Then, the *cro* gene is derepressed, and cro proteins are formed. These proteins then occupy the O_{R3} operator, and turn off in this way the transcription of the *cI* gene (see figure 5.5), allowing its own synthesis. Various kinds of proteins are expressed, and many phage molecules are produced, leading to bacterium death. The reader can consult [142] for more details of this fascinating process. The phage lambda genetic switch is interesting since it provides a complex system involving two negative feedback loops, and is, together with the lac operon, the system where gene regulation was discovered; see, e.g., [132] or [95].

Basically, one should model the stochastic behaviour of this switch using Markov chains by following the random evolution of the number of proteins produced by the *cro* and *cI* genes, and by also taking into account the promoter states, as was done in chapter 1. A stochastic model has been proposed in [7] (see also [150], [92] or [134]). We follow here the authors of [2], by proposing a static model of the **lysogenic mode** based on the occupation of the various operators, using Botzmann-Gibbs free energies.

The λ right operator O_R consists of three sites to which repressor dimers bind cooperatively, thus leading to a system of size $2^3 = 8$ states of the form $n = (n_1, n_2, n_3)$, with $n_i = 0$, 1, reflecting the occupancy of the O_{R1}, O_{R2} and O_{R3} operators. The model of [2] uses three intrinsic binding free energy differences $\triangle H_1$, $\triangle H_2$ and $\triangle H_3$, reflecting binding to the three operator sites in the absence of binding at the others. The reference state is equal to $(0,0,0)$, so that $\triangle H_1 = H(1,0,0) - H(0,0,0)$, $\triangle H_2 = H(0,1,0) - H(0,0,0)$

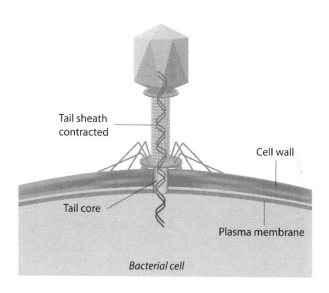

FIGURE 5.3: A phage infecting a bacterium through injection of its DNA into the bacterium genome.

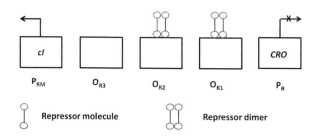

FIGURE 5.4: Transcription of the *cro* gene is turned off when repressor dimers occupy O_{R1}, O_{R2} or both.

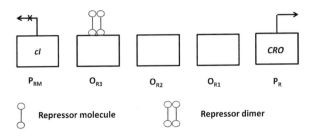

FIGURE 5.5: Transcription of the *cI* gene is turned off when O_{R3} is occupied by a repressor dimer.

and $\triangle H_3 = H(0,0,1) - H(0,0,0)$. Using the notations of section 5.11, one sets

$$K_1 = \exp(-\beta\triangle H_1), \ K_2 = \exp(-\beta\triangle H_2) \text{ and } K_3 = \exp(-\beta\triangle H_3).$$

One admits the following experimental facts:

1. Repressor dimers can bind simultaneously to adjacent operator sites. The related binding free energies are $\triangle H_1 + \triangle H_2 + \triangle H_{12}$ for binding at O_{R1} and O_{R2}, and $\triangle H_2 + \triangle H_3 + \triangle H_{23}$ for binding at O_{R2} and O_{R3}.

2. Cooperative interactions between adjacent bound repressors at O_{R2} and O_{R3} occur only when O_{R1} is vacant.

3. Transcription of the *cro* gene from the right promoter P_R is turned OFF when either O_{R1} or O_{R2} is occupied.

4. A repressor dimer bound to O_{R3} is necessary and sufficient to turn OFF the P_{RM} promoter governing the transcription of the associated gene *cI*.

Cooperative binding is modelled by introducing the free energies $\triangle H_{ij}$, which are the free energy differences between the total free energy to occupy two adjacent sites i and j simultaneously and the sum of the intrinsic binding free energies $\triangle H_i$ and $\triangle H_j$. The Boltzmann weight associated with the binding state $n = (1,1,0)$ is

$$\exp(-\beta\triangle H_{12})\exp(-\beta\triangle H_1)\exp(-\beta\triangle H_2) = \exp(-\beta\triangle H_{12})K_1 K_2,$$

so that the interaction constant c_{12} of section 5.11 is such that

$$c_{12} = \exp(-\beta\triangle H_{12}).$$

One defines c_{23} similarly. We will see in what follows that no pairwise interaction occurs in the configuration $n = (1, 0, 1)$.

Concerning the fully occupied configuration $n = (1, 1, 1)$ (species 8 in table 5.1), the authors of [2] proposed a binding free energy of the form $\triangle H_1 + \triangle H_2 + \triangle H_3 + \triangle H_{12}$, so that cooperative binding only occurs between sites $i = 1$ and $j = 2$. Latter, the authors of [156] proposed a more general model, which is based on the free energy $\triangle H_1 + \triangle H_2 + \triangle H_3 + \triangle H_{123}$, for a new interaction energy H_{123}, as given by species 9 in table 5.1. The numerical values of these binding free energies have been estimated in [2] to be such that $\triangle H_1 = -11.69 \pm 0.03$ kcal, $\triangle H_2 = -10.10 \pm 0.05$ kcal, $\triangle H_3 = -10.09 \pm 0.02$ kcal, $\triangle H_{12} = -1.99 \pm 0.06$ kcal and $\triangle H_{23} = -1.94 \pm 0.06$ kcal.

TABLE 5.1: Free energies associated with the various possible configurations, adapted from [2] and [156].

n	Configuration	Free energy	$\triangle H(n)$ kcal
1	(0,0,0)	Reference state	0
2	(1,0,0)	$\triangle H_1$	-11.7
3	(0,1,0)	$\triangle H_2$	-10.1
4	(0,0,1)	$\triangle H_3$	-10.1
5	(1,1,0)	$\triangle H_1 + \triangle H_2 + \triangle H_{12}$	-23.8
6	(1,0,1)	$\triangle H_1 + \triangle H_3$	-21.8
7	(0,1,1)	$\triangle H_2 + \triangle H_3 + \triangle H_{23}$	-22.2
8	(1,1,1)	$\triangle H_1 + \triangle H_2 + \triangle H_3 + \triangle H_{12}$	-33.9
9	(1,1,1)	$\triangle H_1 + \triangle H_2 + \triangle H_3 + \triangle H_{123}$	

The probability of any configuration n is then given by

$$\pi_\beta(n) = \frac{\exp(-\beta \triangle H(n))[R]^{|n|}}{\sum_{n'} \exp(-\beta \triangle H(n'))[R]^{|n'|}},$$

where $[R]$ denotes the concentration of free repressor dimers, and where the free energy differences $\triangle H(n) = H(n) - H(0, 0, 0)$ are provided in table 5.1. The probability that the promoter P_{RM} is OFF is given by the probability that operator O_{R3} is occupied:

$$\pi_\beta(P_{RM} \text{ is OFF}) = \pi_\beta(4) + \pi_\beta(6) + \pi_\beta(7) + \pi_\beta(8)$$

(see table 5.1 and figure 5.6), while the probability that the promoter P_R is OFF is given by

$$\pi_\beta(P_R \text{ is OFF}) = \pi_\beta(2) + \pi_\beta(3) + \pi_\beta(5) + \pi_\beta(6) + \pi_\beta(7) + \pi_\beta(8).$$

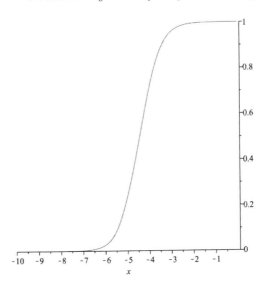

FIGURE 5.6: Plot of the probability $\pi_\beta(P_{RM}$ is OFF$)$ versus log repressor concentration.

Boltzmann machine structure

It turns out that the total free energy function $\triangle H(n)$ can be expressed using the Boltzmann machine model given in example 5.3.3, with $S = \{1, 2, 3\}$; see (5.12). The intrinsic free energies $\triangle H_i$ are associated with the singletons $\{1\}$, $\{2\}$ and $\{3\}$. This leads to the three terms

$$\triangle H_1 n_1 + \triangle H_2 n_2 + \triangle H_3 n_3.$$

Next, one can use rule (2) to add a cooperative term of the form

$$\triangle H_{23} n_2 n_3 (1 - n_1),$$

which takes into account the restriction on the vacancy of operator O_{R1}. For the Boltzmann machine model, this yields the two terms

$$\triangle H_{23} n_2 n_3,$$

for $S' = \{2, 3\}$, and

$$-\triangle H_{23} n_1 n_2 n_3,$$

for the subset $S' = S = \{1, 2, 3\}$, a three-body interaction term. Finally, the first rule (1) permits the introduction of the last term

$$\triangle H_{12} n_1 n_2,$$

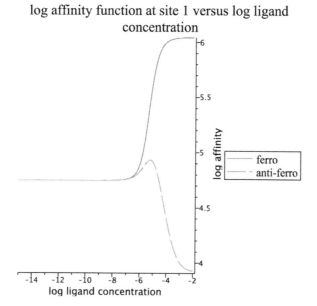

log affinity function at site 1 versus log ligand concentration

FIGURE 5.7: Plot of the log affinity function $^v K_1$ at site 1 versus the log ligand concentration. The curves correspond to the two values $\triangle H_{123} = -5$ and $\triangle H_{123} = -0.01$. When $\triangle H_{123} = -5$, the Boltzmann machine has only ferromagnetic coupling coefficients, while when $\triangle H_{123} = -0.01$, the three-body interaction term is anti-ferromagnetic. These pictures lead to positive and negative cooperativity at site 1.

for $S' = \{1, 2\}$, so that

$$\triangle H(n) = \triangle H_1 n_1 + \triangle H_2 n_2 + \triangle H_3 n_3 + \triangle H_{12} n_1 n_2$$
$$+ \triangle H_{23} n_2 n_3 - \triangle H_{23} n_1 n_2 n_3,$$

$n_i = 0, 1$, which is a Boltzmann machine model with up to three-body interactions. Note that the term $-\triangle H_{23} n_1 n_2 n_3$ is anti-ferromagnetic (see figure 5.7). If one considers the more recent model of [156] by opting for species 9 instead of species 8, the related energy function $\triangle H(n)$ is

$$\triangle H(n) = \triangle H_1 n_1 + \triangle H_2 n_2 + \triangle H_3 n_3 + \triangle H_{12} n_1 n_2 + \triangle H_{23} n_2 n_3$$
$$+ (\triangle H_{123} - \triangle H_{12} - \triangle H_{23}) n_1 n_2 n_3,$$

which is again a Boltzmann machine model with up to three-body interactions.

Chapter 6

Kinetics of binding processes

Transcription in eukaryotes involves complex biological processes, like transcription factors (TF) binding and chromatin remodelling, which are dynamical in nature. The preceding sections focus on chemical equilibrium, where the steady state is described by some probability measure π, as described in section 5.2. We assume in this section that $\pi = \pi_\beta$ is a Gibbs-Boltzmann distribution associated with some free energy function H. These distributions should coincide with steady state distributions of Markov chains describing chemical kinetics. Cooperativity is quite often introduced using dynamical arguments. We hence focus on basic Markov chains describing binding processes. Assume that the binding process is such that only one ligand molecule can bind per unit time (sequential binding), that is, suppose that the possible transitions are of the form, for $i = 1, \cdots, N$,

$$n = (n_1, \cdots, n_{i-1}, 0, n_{i+1}, \cdots, n_N) \longrightarrow n' = (n_1, \cdots, n_{i-1}, 1, n_{i+1}, \cdots, n_N),$$

which corresponds to the binding of a new ligand molecule at site i, or, for dissociation at site i,

$$n = (n_1, \cdots, n_{i-1}, 1, n_{i+1}, \cdots, n_N) \longrightarrow n' = (n_1, \cdots, n_{i-1}, 0, n_{i+1}, \cdots, n_N).$$

We look for transition rates ensuring that the steady state is π_β. Let $q_{nn'}$ and $q_{n'n}$ be the rates associated with these transitions, which should satisfy the detailed balance equation (2.11)

$$\pi_\beta(n)q_{nn'} = \pi_\beta(n')q_{n'n}.$$

In this situation,

$$\frac{\pi_\beta(n')}{\pi_\beta(n)} = \frac{v^{|n'|}}{v^{|n|}} \frac{\exp(-\beta H(n'))}{\exp(-\beta H(n))} = \frac{q_{nn'}}{q_{n'n}}.$$

For the binding of a new ligand molecule, $|n'| = |n| + 1$, so that this last condition becomes

$$\frac{\pi_\beta(n')}{\pi_\beta(n)} = v\frac{\exp(-\beta H(n'))}{\exp(-\beta H(n))} = \frac{q_{nn'}}{q_{n'n}}.$$

A possible choice for the binding rates is

$$q_{nn'} = v \exp(-\beta(H(n') - H(n))), \text{ and, for dissociation, } q_{n'n} = 1. \quad (6.1)$$

One can find many physical arguments to validate such transition rates. The reader can consult [125] for interesting examples. Notice that Metropolis chains based on the free energy function $\bar{H}(n) = H(n) - |n| \ln(v)/\beta$ are also good candidates; see (2.18). When $H(n) = V(|n|)$ for some function V (see example 5.3.1), one can forget the microscopic world and focus on the state space $\tilde{\Lambda} = \{0, 1, \cdots, N\}$ giving the possible number of bound sites. In this setting, the natural binding probability is

$$\tilde{\pi}_\beta(k) = \frac{\binom{N}{k} v^k \exp(-\beta V(k))}{\sum_{k=0}^{N} \binom{N}{k} v^k \exp(-\beta V(k))}. \quad (6.2)$$

Let us denote by $(MX)_k$ the state where exactly k ligand molecules are bound on the macromolecule. Consider the reaction

$$(MX)_k + X \underset{\kappa_-^{k+1}}{\overset{\kappa_+^k}{\longleftrightarrow}} (MX)_{k+1}. \quad (6.3)$$

The binding rate κ_+^k and the dissociation rate κ_-^{k+1} should be such that

$$\tilde{\pi}_\beta(k)\kappa_+^k = \tilde{\pi}_\beta(k+1)\kappa_-^{k+1}, \quad (6.4)$$

which is the detailed balance equation (2.11). The reader can check that

$$\kappa_+^k = v(N-k) \exp(-\beta(V(k+1) - V(k))) \text{ and } \kappa_-^{k+1} = (k+1)$$

satisfy this last requirement. Notice that these rates make sense, since, for example, the factor in front of the exponential in κ_+^k takes into account the ligand concentration v and a combinatorial factor accounting for the fact that a new ligand molecule can bind at $(N-k)$ sites, which are ligand free. The related equilibrium constants are defined by

$$K^k = \frac{\kappa_+^k}{\kappa_-^k} = \frac{v(N-k)}{k+1} \exp(-\beta(V(k+1) - V(k))).$$

6.1 A mathematical model of eukaryotic gene activation

The Epstein-Barr virus (EBV) transactivator Zebra is an important TF which synergistically enhances transcription, and provides an interesting

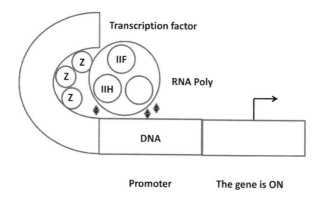

FIGURE 6.1: Zebra molecules bind to DNA on specific sites. The general transcription machinery then binds to these Zebra molecules cooperatively. The complex then interacts chemically with the promoter, leading to gene activation.

paradigm for studying eukaryotic regulation. We consider a mathematical model proposed in [184], which illustrates well regulation with TF. This model is based on previous studies in different contexts by [2]. Similar models were then developed in [181] and [27].

Zebra stimulates transcription by interacting with parts of the general transcription machinery. We will not enter into the details of these complex processes, but illustrate how principles from thermodynamics can help in understanding regulation in this setting. The reader is invited to see [184] to get all the biological and biochemical information. Their *in vitro* model consists in a system composed of human transcription extracts, of recombined Zebra and of templates containing multiple binding sites upstream of a core promoter. The mathematical model is divided into four main steps, each of them corresponding to a well established phase; see figure 6.2.

Binding of Zebra molecules to DNA

In this first step, Zebra molecules bind to DNA on multiple sites upstream of a core promoter. The chemical reactions corresponding to these binding events are described using binding free energy $\triangle z < 0$, which gives the amount of free energy needed for a Zebra molecule to interact chemically with a given binding site. These energies can be calculated precisely, using well established methods from biochemistry. In this first step, the model assumes that these binding events are statistically independent, that is, the fact that some Zebra molecule is bound to some site i is independent of what happens at a different site $j \neq i$. In this case, this binding process does not act cooperatively. Let us suppose that the number of binding sites is given by N. Let $[Z]$ be the concentration of Zebra molecules. S_k^z represents the event that k binding sites are occupied by Zebra molecules, and $[S_k^z]$ denotes the related concentration.

$$S_k^z + Z \longleftrightarrow S_{k+1}^z \qquad (6.5)$$

models the reaction where a new Zebra molecule is being bound to DNA given that the number of bound sites is k. The authors of [184] proposed the following detailed balance equation:

$$(N - k)e^{-\beta \triangle z}[S_k^z][Z] = (k + 1)[S_{k+1}^z], \qquad (6.6)$$

where $\beta = 1/T$, T is the temperature, and where the exponential form of the transition rate is *Arrehnius law*. The factor $(N - k)$ is a combinatorial coefficient related to the fact that a new Zebra molecule can bind to $(N - k)$ sites when k binding sites are already occupied. The mass action principle indicates that the equilibrium constant K^k should be related to the concentrations according to the identity

$$K^k = \frac{[S_{k+1}^z]}{[S_k^z][Z]}.$$

Using Arrehenius law to write $\kappa_f = \exp(-\beta E_f)$ and $\kappa_r = \exp(-\beta E_r)$, for activation energies E_f and E_r such that $E_f - E_r = \triangle z$, one can see formula (6.6) as expressing the transitions $(k \rightarrow k+1)$ and $(k+1 \rightarrow k)$ of a Markov chain of transition rates $[Z](N-k)\kappa_f/\kappa_r = [Z](N-k)\exp(-\beta \triangle z)$ and $(k+1)$; see (6.1). More precisely, let $[S_{\text{tot}}]$ be the total template concentration. One can rewrite (6.6) as the reversibility condition (2.11) (see also (6.4)):

$$\frac{[S_k^z]}{[S_{\text{tot}}]}(N - k)[Z]e^{-\beta(E_f - E_r)} = \frac{[S_{k+1}^z]}{[S_{\text{tot}}]}(k + 1).$$

When the number of templates, of Zebra molecules and of factors is large, and when statistical equilibrium is attained, the ratio $[S_k^z]/[S_{\text{tot}}]$ should correspond to the steady state distribution of this stochastic process. This Markov chain is a birth and death process of birth and death rates $\lambda_k = (N-k)\exp(-\beta \triangle z)[Z]$ and $\nu_k = k$, and of invariant measure $\tilde{\pi}_\beta^z$ (see example 2.2.3)

$$\tilde{\pi}_\beta^z(k) = \frac{\prod_{l=0}^{k-1} \lambda_l \prod_{l=k+1}^{N} \nu_l}{\sum_{k=0}^{N} \prod_{l=0}^{k-1} \lambda_l \prod_{l=k+1}^{N} \nu_l} = \frac{\binom{N}{k}e^{-\beta k \triangle z}[Z]^k}{I_z(N)},$$

where the normalization constant $I_z(N)$ is

$$I_z(N) = \sum_{k=0}^{N} \binom{N}{k} e^{-\beta k \triangle z} [Z]^k = (1 + [Z] e^{-\beta \triangle z})^N.$$

Note that this probability measure is (6.2) with $V(k) = k\triangle z$. Hence, the distribution of bound Zebra molecules is binomial $\mathrm{Bi}(N, p)$ with parameter of success $p = [Z] \exp(-\beta \triangle z)/(1 + [Z] \exp(-\beta \triangle z))$. In the microscopic version of this model, the N occupations binary random variables corresponding to the N binding sites are i.i.d. Bernoulli of parameter p, and the model is thus not cooperative.

Binding of Zebra molecules to the general transcription machinery

Let us suppose that $k \leq N$ DNA binding sites are occupied by Zebra molecules at steady state. These bound activators can also bind to the various factors composing the general transcription machinery, which is composed of RNA polymerase II (polII), of a set of TF, and of a class of co-activator proteins (see [184] for more details on the related biochemistry). Two possible pathways can be considered for the assembly of the transcription complex: a holoenzyme pathway where some of these factors are pre-assembled into a complex, and a model where these factors are free in solution but where a nucleation process begins after the recruitment of one or several key transcription factors, which leads to the assembly of the transcription machinery on DNA.

The main difference with the previous step is that the binding of factors to the set of bound Zebra is **cooperative**: a factor can bind to a bound Zebra molecule with some interaction free energy $\triangle f < 0$, but, in addition, the binding of one factor to a Zebra molecule will enhance the binding of the other factors. This can be the effect of **conformational changes** resulting from the binding of the first factors (as, for example, isomerization, see [184]).

Let $\triangle g < 0$ be an additional free energy accounting for this cooperative effect. In what follows, we denote by $S_k^z Z_m^F$ the biochemical state where k sites are occupied by Zebra molecules, and where m of them are also bound or interact with components of the transcription machinery. Due to the cooperative effect, one must distinguish the cases $m = 0$ and $m \geq 1$. The analogue of (6.5) becomes

$$S_k^z Z_m^F + \mathrm{F} \longleftrightarrow S_k^z Z_{m+1}^F, \quad m = 0, 1, \cdots, k, \tag{6.7}$$

and the related detailed balance equations are hence of the form

$$ke^{-\beta\triangle f}[S_k^z Z_0^F][F] = [S_k^z Z_1^F], \ m = 0, \tag{6.8}$$

$$(k-m)e^{-\beta(\triangle f+\triangle g)}[S_k^z Z_m^F][F] = (m+1)[S_k^z Z_{m+1}^F], \ m = 1, \cdots, k. \tag{6.9}$$

Intuitively, positive cooperative binding follows from the fact that $e^{-\beta\triangle g} > 1$ since $\triangle g < 0$. One can check that the unique invariant probability measure is, for fixed k,

$$\tilde{\pi}_\beta^{k,F}(m) = \frac{\binom{k}{m}[F]^m e^{-\beta m\triangle f} e^{-(m-1)\beta\triangle g}}{I_F(k)}, \quad \text{when } m \geq 1,$$

and

$$\tilde{\pi}_\beta^{k,F}(0) = \frac{1}{I_F(k)},$$

when $m = 0$, where the normalization constant $I_F(k)$ is

$$\begin{aligned} I_F(k) &= 1 + \sum_{m=1}^{k} \binom{k}{m}[F]^m e^{-\beta m\triangle f} e^{-(m-1)\beta\triangle g} \\ &= 1 + \exp(\beta\triangle g)(1 + [F]\exp(-\beta(\triangle f + \triangle g)))^k - 1). \end{aligned}$$

The reader is invited to check cooperativity in exercise 6.1.1.

Tethering of the Zebra factor complex to the core promoter

The Zebra general factor complex can bind to the core promoter with some interaction free energy $\triangle p$, which measures the affinity of the promoter for the complex. The authors of [184] also consider a synergistic interaction to take into account isomerization or conformational changes which occur when m is large enough, here when $m > 1$, which enhance transcription. Let $\triangle q$ be a free energy modelling this synergistic interaction. The associated reaction is represented by the following scheme:

$$S_k^z Z_m^F + P \longleftrightarrow S_k^z Z_m^F P, \ m = 1, \cdots, k, \tag{6.10}$$

for fixed values of k and m, where P is a symbol representing the promoter. The related detailed balance equations are

$$[S_k^z Z_m^F]e^{-\beta\triangle p} = [S_k^z Z_m^F P], \ m = 1, \tag{6.11}$$

and

$$[S_k^z Z_m^F]e^{-\beta(\triangle p+\triangle q)} = [S_k^z Z_m^F P], \ m > 1. \tag{6.12}$$

It is perhaps useful to consider in more detail the above chemical reactions: consider the Arrehenius law to write the forward rate $\kappa_f = \exp(-\beta \triangle_{01})$ and backward rate $\kappa_r = 1$, where $\triangle_{01} = \triangle p$ when $m = 1$ and $\triangle_{01} = \triangle p + \triangle q$ when $m > 1$. The gene is ON ($\mathcal{O}_1$) when the Zebra general factor complex is bound to the promoter, and OFF($\mathcal{O}_0$) otherwise. This reaction can be seen as a two state Markov chain of transitions

$$\mathcal{O}_0 \underset{\kappa_r}{\overset{\kappa_f}{\longleftrightarrow}} \mathcal{O}_1,$$

of forward rate κ_f and backward rate κ_r. The steady state distribution $\pi_\beta^{(m,k)}$ is

$$\pi_\beta^{(m,k)}(\text{ON}) = \frac{\kappa_f}{\kappa_f + \kappa_r}.$$

Using the distinction between cases $m = 1$ and $m > 1$, one gets the formula

$$\pi_\beta^{(m,k)}(\text{ON}) = \begin{cases} \frac{e^{-\beta \triangle p}}{1 + e^{-\beta \triangle p}} & \text{when } m = 1, \\ \frac{e^{-\beta(\triangle p + \triangle q)}}{1 + e^{-\beta(\triangle p + \triangle q)}} & \text{when } m > 1. \end{cases}$$

The transcription rate $T(\beta, [Z], [F])$ is obtained by averaging this probability, which depends on both m and k, with respect to the probability measures $\tilde{\pi}_\beta^z$ and $\tilde{\pi}_\beta^F$:

$$T(\beta, [Z], [F]) = \sum_{k=1}^{N} \tilde{\pi}_\beta^z(k) \sum_{m=1}^{k} \tilde{\pi}_\beta^{k,F}(m) \pi_\beta^{(m,k)}(\text{ON}). \tag{6.13}$$

This model reproduces well experimental data, see [184]. Figure 6.2 shows the effect of cooperativity on transcription rates, when modelled in this way.

Exercise 6.1.1 Assume that k Zebra molecules are bound to DNA, and consider the probability measure $\tilde{\pi}_\beta^{k,F}$, which models the binding of factors to the set of bound Zebra molecules. Let n_i, $i = 1, \cdots, k$ be the occupation variables associated with the k Zebra molecules.

- Show that the probability measure corresponding to $\tilde{\pi}_\beta^{k,F}$ is

$$\pi_\beta^{k,F}(n_1, \cdots, n_k) = \frac{\exp(-\beta V(|n|))}{Z_\beta^{k,F}},$$

where $V(0) = 0$ and $V(m) = m(\triangle f + \triangle g) - \triangle g$ when $m \geq 1$, and where $Z_\beta^{k,F}$ is the associated partition function.

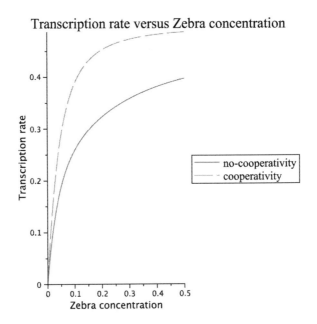

FIGURE 6.2: Plot of the transcription rate $T(\beta, [Z], [F])$ versus Zebra concentration $[Z]$. The parameters are chosen as in [184]. One sees the effect of adding cooperative free energy terms ($\triangle g < 0$).

- Show that

$$\text{Cov}_{\pi_\beta^{k,F}}(n_i, n_j) > 0, \quad \forall i \neq j,$$

if and only if $\triangle g < 0$. In this case, the binding of the various factors to the k bound Zebra molecules exhibits positive cooperativity.

6.2   Steady state distribution of more general binding processes

Section 5.12 focuses on models where a free energy function governs the statistical equilibrium of binding processes. In many situations, however, chemical reactions are described by transition rates which follow well known laws like Arrhenius law. The so-called Eyring model [69] assumes that transitions from state x to state y are of the form

$$q_{xy} = \frac{\kappa_B T}{h} \exp(\frac{\triangle_{xy} S}{R}) \exp(-\frac{\triangle_{xy} H}{RT}),$$

where κ_B is Boltzmann's constant, R is the perfect gas constant, h is Planck's constant, and where $\triangle_{xy} H$ and $\triangle S_{xy}$ are, respectively, the activation enthalpies and entropies. Setting $\beta = T^{-1}$, one can use theorem 2.2.4 to check that the steady state distribution is not given by a Gibbs distribution in general.

Section 5.13 describes a model of equilibrium of λ phage repressor regulation, where the operator occupancy is described using the notion of Boltzmann machines for some experimentally deduced energy function H. This model assumes that the repressor concentration $[R]$ is fixed, so that $[R]$ becomes a natural parameter of the statistical model. In reality, $[R]$ fluctuates randomly as a function of time, and its expression level strongly depends on operator occupancy (double negative feedback). Hence one should consider an extended model of random variables given by $n = (n_1, n_2, n_3)$ and by the random number of cI and Cro protein dimers. The steady state distribution of this enlarged Markov chain is difficult to obtain in closed form, and, for example, using the matrix tree theorem, one should be able to check that it does not correspond exactly to a Gibbs measure. The interested reader can consult [7], where a stochastic model of this bistable switch is provided.

Chapters 7 and 8 focus on genetic switches described by dynamics that do not fall in the framework of chapter 6. One can, however, study the related binding probabilities using tools developed in section 5.12.

Chapter 7

Transcription factor binding at nucleosomal DNA

DNA is in intimate contact with protein complexes called nucleosomes, which can in many instances prevent transcription factor (TF) binding by rendering the TF binding site non-accessible. We present here models which explain how indirect cooperative effects emerge from the competition between nucleosomes and TF. We follow essentially the works of [130], [155], [140] and [146], but recall that these questions are still under active debate in molecular biology.

7.1 Competition between nucleosomes and TF

We present here the simplest of the models given in [155] and [146], which focus on the competition for binding between nucleosomes and TF. Let s be a DNA sequence of length L where TF can bind. The binding free energy is often assumed to be of the form

$$\triangle H = \sum_{k=0}^{L} \sum_{b \in \{A,T,G,C\}} S(b,k)\varepsilon_{kb}, \tag{7.1}$$

where $S(b,k) = 1$ if the kth base of the sequence s is b, and where $S(b,k) = 0$ otherwise, and where the ε_{kb} are the site specific binding free energies. This additive model was presented in [17], and was then used in bioinformatics for predicting protein-DNA binding sites; see, e.g., [164], [26] and [15]. Suppose that there is a single binding site of associated sequence s. The rate function is proportional to the probability that the binding site is occupied by a TF:

$$T_1(\beta, v) = \langle |n| \rangle_{\pi_\beta} = \pi_\beta(n_1 = 1) = \frac{v \exp(-\beta \triangle H)}{1 + v \exp(-\beta \triangle H)},$$

where v denotes the TF concentration. When nucleosomes are also considered, the state space is enlarged to take into account the states where some histone is bound (the state $\mathcal{O}_0$) or the case where the DNA is naked, that is, is free of nucleosomes, denoted by $\mathcal{O}_1$ in what follows. In this second model, the rate function becomes

$$T_2(\beta, v) = \frac{S_A v \exp(-\beta \triangle H)}{1 + S_A v \exp(-\beta \triangle H) + S_N},$$

where S_N and S_A are combinatorial weights associated with the nucleosome positioning. The authors of [146] studied the effect of adding nucleosomes to the rate function T: for a given level t, consider the equation

$$t = T_1(\beta, v_1) = T_2(\beta, v_2).$$

A computation shows that

$$v_2 = v_1 \frac{S_A + S_N}{S_A},$$

so that the plot of the rate function T_2 is essentially a shift of the plot of T_1. This simple model was then extended by adding various regulation mechanisms. The authors of [146] explained in this way how repressor complexes like nucleosomes can induce obligate cooperativity.

7.2   Nucleosome-mediated cooperativity between TF

The cooperative effects described in section 5.13 were induced by direct interactions between repressor molecules. The model of eukaryotic gene activation provided in section 6.1 introduced cooperativity through conformational changes. The recent models of [130], [146] and [155] propose mechanisms leading to cooperativity in an indirect way, or as a result of the competition between TF binding and nucleosome positioning. These models consider transcription factor binding sites (TFBS) which can be occupied by histones; see figure 7.1. When bound, this nucleosomal DNA may prevent the binding of TF to the TFBS. In [140], synergistic binding of two nearby TF is possible: the first bound TF induces a partial unwrapping of the nucleosomal DNA which favors the binding of the second TF.

In [130], a model is proposed which aims at describing the stochastic evolution of such systems: the histone can be bound or unbound. The first situation

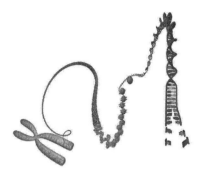

FIGURE 7.1: Nucleosomal DNA.

will be described as the OFF state $\mathcal{O}_0$, while the case where the DNA is naked will be represented as an ON state $\mathcal{O}_1$. The rate of switching between these two states will be denoted by g for the OFF/ON transition, and by κ for the ON/OFF transition. We use these notations since the mathematical model has the same form as the model considered for the self-regulated gene; see chapter 1. Let $L = g/\kappa$. Assume that the sequence contains N TFBS, and let us denote by n_i, $i = 1, \cdots, N$ the related occupation random variables, of ligation number $|n|$. The state space of the Markov chain is composed of pairs (k, y) where $0 \leq k \leq N$ models ligation, and where the binary variable y is such that $y = 0$ when the histone is bound and $y = 1$ otherwise.

Consider the macroscopic description of the binding process, as described by (6.3). In this setting, $(MX)_k$ denotes the state where exactly k TF molecules are bound on the DNA sequence. The variable X represents TF, and v gives the related concentration. The author of [130] assumes that conformational changes leading to nucleosomal or accessible DNA only occur when the DNA is free of TF. The stochastic change of the ligation number is described by the relation

$$(MX)_k + X \underset{\kappa_{-,y}^{k+1}}{\overset{\kappa_{+,y}^{k}}{\rightleftarrows}} (MX)_{k+1}, \ 0 \leq k \leq N-1, \mathcal{O}_0 \underset{\kappa}{\overset{g}{\rightleftarrows}} \mathcal{O}_1, \ k = 0, \qquad (7.2)$$

where

$$\kappa_{+,y}^{k} = v(N-k)\mu_1 \text{ and } \kappa_{-,y}^{k} = k,$$

when $y = 1$, and

$$\kappa_{+,y}^{k} = v(N-k)\mu_0 \text{ and } \kappa_{-,y}^{k} = k,$$

when $y = 0$, where we suppose that $\mu_0 < \mu_1$ since the TF binding rates are diminished in the OFF state. The last reaction

$$\mathcal{O}_0 \xleftrightarrow[\kappa]{g} \mathcal{O}_1, \ k = 0,$$

indicates that the switch between the states $\mathcal{O}_0$ (nucleosomal DNA) and $\mathcal{O}_1$ (the site is nucleosome-free) can occur only when the binding site is free of TF. The same kind of constraint is imposed in the Monod-Wyman-Changeux model of allosteric regulation (see [131]), which is known to yield strong cooperativity in the Hill sense. The author of [130] computes the Hill coefficient using several kinds of approximations, by defining the statistical weights $w(k,0)$ and $w(k,1)$, for the OFF and ON states,

$$w(k,0) = \binom{N}{k}(\mu_0 v)^k \text{ and } w(k,1) = \binom{N}{k}(\mu_1 v)^k,$$

of partition function

$$Z_{\text{tot}} = \sum_{k=0}^{N}(w(k,0) + Lw(k,1)) = Z_0 + LZ_1,$$

where

$$Z_0 = (1 + \mu_0 v)^N \text{ and } Z_1 = (1 + \mu_1 v)^N.$$

These weights are then used to define a probability measure λ as

$$\lambda(k,1) = \frac{Lw(k,1)}{Z_{\text{tot}}}, \tag{7.3}$$

for the ON state $\mathcal{O}_1$ with k bound TF, and

$$\lambda(k,0) = \frac{w(k,0)}{Z_{\text{tot}}} \tag{7.4}$$

for the OFF state.

Recalling that there is a transition between the OFF and ON states only when no TF is bound, the reader can notice that λ is nothing but the invariant probability measure of a birth and death process evolving in a segment composed of three pieces (see figure 7.2): the first piece corresponds to the sequential binding or unbinding of TF in the ON state, the second piece is associated with the switching between the ON and OFF states and vice versa, while the last piece is the sequential binding and unbinding of TF in the OFF state.

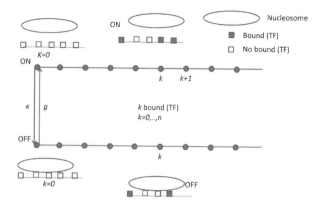

FIGURE 7.2: Transition diagram associated the model (7.2): the system can switch between the accessible and nucleosomal DNA only when no TF is bound on DNA.

We next focus on the number of bound TF in either the ON or OFF state: let

$$\omega(k) = \lambda(k,0) + \lambda(k,1), \ k = 0, 1, \cdots, N.$$

The associated mean ligation number is (see section 5.2)

$$\langle |n| \rangle_\omega = \sum_{k=0}^{N} k\omega(k) = \sum_{k=0}^{N} k(\lambda(k,0) + \lambda(k,1)).$$

Let

$$\eta_H(v) = \frac{\mathrm{d} \ln(\frac{\langle |n| \rangle_\omega}{N - \langle |n| \rangle_\omega})}{\mathrm{d} \ln(v)} = \frac{\mathrm{Var}_\omega(|n|)}{N\frac{\langle |n| \rangle_\omega}{N}(1 - \frac{\langle |n| \rangle_\omega}{N})},$$

be the Hill coefficient. When $\mu_0 = 0$, the Hill coefficient is

$$\eta_H(v) = \frac{L(1 + \mu_1 v)^N + 1 + N\mu_1 v}{L(1 + \mu_1 v)^N + 1 + \mu_1 v}.$$

When, moreover,

$$L = g/\kappa \ll 1,$$

so that the switch strongly favours the OFF state, the author of [130] obtained that the Hill coefficient is such that

$$\sup_v \eta_H(v) = N\frac{v^*}{1 + v^*},$$

for some critical concentration v^*, with

$$v^* \sim \frac{1}{(L(N-1))^{\frac{1}{N}}} - 1.$$

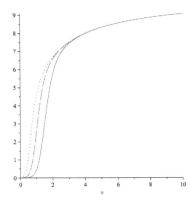

FIGURE 7.3: Plots of the mean ligation number $\langle |n|\rangle_\omega/N$, for $N = 10$, $\mu_0 = 0$, $\mu_1 = 1$, $g = 0.001$ and $L = 0.0001$ (solid line), $L = 0.001$ (long dash) and $L = 0.01$ (dots). The curve has an S-shape for low values of L.

The system is thus strongly cooperative for large N; see figure 7.3.

At low concentrations, the empty configuration with no bound TF has a large probability while the other configurations have small probabilities; see figure 7.4. At intermediate concentrations, the probability distribution becomes bimodal with a high variance; see figure 7.5. At large concentrations, the distribution is essentially supported by configurations having a large number of bound sites; see figure 7.6. Figure 7.7 shows that the variance is maximal for some intermediate value of v. Recalling that the Hill coefficient $\eta_H(v)$ is directly related to the variance of the ligation number (see above or (5.17)), one understands why there is a critical intermediate value of v leading to the maximum of $\eta_H(v)$, which is proportional to N in the present situation; see figure 7.8. This shows the surprising result that, according to this model, the competition between TF binding and nucleosome positioning leads to strong positive cooperativity since the Hill coefficient is asymptotically linear in the number N of TFBS.

However, one may wonder what is the situation when conformational changes leading to nucleosomal DNA or nucleosome free DNA occur even when TF are bound for arbitrary TF binding configurations; see figure 7.9.

Nucleosome-mediated cooperativity: two different models

We consider the stochastic process $(m(t), y(t))$, $t \geq 0$, where $m(t)$ denotes the ligation number at time t, and where $y(t) = 1$ means that the histone is

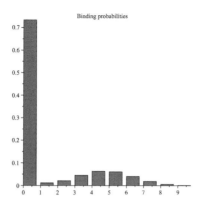

FIGURE 7.4: Plot of $\omega(k)$, $k = 0, \ldots, N$, $N = 10$ (see (7.3) and (7.4)), when $\mu_0 = 0.001$, $\mu_1 = 1$, $g = 0.001$, $\kappa = 1$ and $v = 0.8$. At low concentration, the state with no bound TF has a high probability while the other configurations have low probabilities.

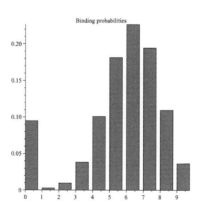

FIGURE 7.5: Plot of $\omega(k)$, $k = 0, \ldots, N$, $N = 10$, when $\mu_0 = 0.001$, $\mu_1 = 1$, $g = 0.001$, $\kappa = 1$ and $v = 1.5$. At intermediate concentration, the probability distribution is bimodal and has a large variance.

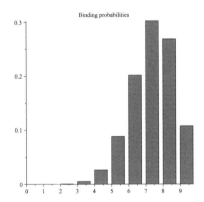

FIGURE 7.6: Plot of $\omega(k)$, $k = 0, \ldots, N$, $N = 10$, when $\mu_0 = 0.001$, $\mu_1 = 1$, $g = 0.001$, $\kappa = 1$ and $v = 4$. At high concentration, the states with large numbers of bound sites dominate.

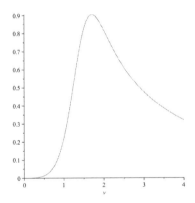

FIGURE 7.7: Plot of the ligation number variance when $N = 10$, $\mu_0 = 0$, $\mu_1 = 1$, $g = 0.001$, $\kappa = 1$ and $L = 0.01$. One observes that the variance attains its maximal value for some intermediate concentration v.

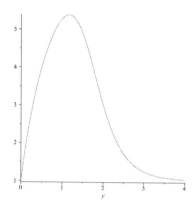

FIGURE 7.8: Plot of the Hill exponent $\eta_H(v)$ when $N = 10$, $\mu_0 = 0$, $\mu_1 = 1$, $g = 0.001$, $\kappa = 1$ and $L = 0.01$.

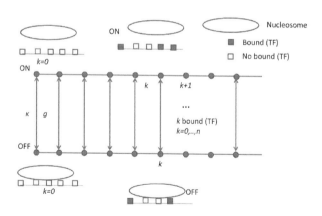

FIGURE 7.9: Transition diagram associated with the model given by (7.5): the system can switch between the accessible and nucleosomal DNA independently of the number of bound (TF).

not bound, which corresponds to the ON state. The set of chemical reactions

$$(MX)_k + X \underset{\kappa_{-,y}^{k+1}}{\overset{\kappa_{+,y}^{k}}{\rightleftarrows}} (MX)_{k+1}, \quad \mathcal{O}_0 \underset{\kappa}{\overset{g}{\rightleftarrows}} \mathcal{O}_1, \tag{7.5}$$

describes the transition rates of the Markov chain $(m(t), y(t))$: let

$$P_{k,0}(t) = P(m(t) = k; \; y(t) = 0) \text{ and } P_{k,1}(t) = P(m(t) = k; \; y(t) = 1).$$

The master equation describing the time evolution of these two sets of probabilities is

$$
\begin{aligned}
\frac{\mathrm{d}P_{k,0}(t)}{\mathrm{d}t} &= v\mu_0(N - k + 1)P_{k-1,0}(t) + (k + 1)P_{k+1,0}(t) + \kappa P_{k,1}(t) \\
&\quad - P_{k,0}(t)(g + k + v\mu_0(N - k)), \\
\frac{\mathrm{d}P_{k,1}(t)}{\mathrm{d}t} &= v\mu_1(N - k + 1)P_{k-1,1}(t) + (k + 1)P_{k+1,1}(t) + gP_{k,0}(t) \\
&\quad - P_{k,1}(t)(\kappa + k + v\mu_1(N - k)).
\end{aligned}
$$

The steady state can be found using the method of transfer matrices (see section A.3), since the present mathematical setting is similar to the mathematical model of chapter 1. We opt here for a more direct approach, using differential equations for the mean ligation numbers. Let us denote by $\tilde{\pi}$ the unique steady state distribution of this Markov chain, which is such that

$$\tilde{\pi}_{k,0} = \lim_{t \to \infty} P_{k,0}(t) \text{ and } \tilde{\pi}_{k,1} = \lim_{t \to \infty} P_{k,1}(t).$$

Recalling that the Hill coefficient is defined using the mean ligation number $\langle |n| \rangle_{\tilde{\pi}}$, we consider the functions

$$E_0(t) = \sum_{k=1}^{N} k P_{k,0}(t), \quad E_1(t) = \sum_{k=1}^{N} k P_{k,1}(t) \text{ and } E(t) = E_0(t) + E_1(t).$$

The mean ligation number is then

$$\langle |n| \rangle_{\tilde{\pi}} = \sum_{k=1}^{N} k(\tilde{\pi}_{k,0} + \tilde{\pi}_{k,1}) = E(\infty).$$

The related master equation yields through direct computation that

$$
\begin{aligned}
\frac{\mathrm{d}E_0(t)}{\mathrm{d}t} &= \kappa E_1(t) + v\mu_0(N P_{OFF}(t) - E_0(t)) - E_0(t) - gE_0(t), \\
\frac{\mathrm{d}E_1(t)}{\mathrm{d}t} &= gE_0(t) + v\mu_1(N P_{ON}(t) - E_1(t)) - E_1(t) - \kappa E_1(t),
\end{aligned}
$$

where $P_{OFF}(t) = \sum_k P_{k,0}(t)$ and $P_{ON}(t) = \sum_k P_{k,1}(t)$ are such that

$$P_{OFF}(\infty) = \frac{\kappa}{\kappa + g} \text{ and } P_{ON}(\infty) = \frac{g}{\kappa + g}.$$

The above system yields that

$$E_0(\infty) = vN \frac{\kappa(g\mu_1 + \mu_0(1 + \kappa + v\mu_1))}{(g + \kappa)(1 + v(\kappa\mu_0 + (g + v\mu_0)\mu_1) + (g + \kappa + v(\mu_0 + \mu_1)))},$$

with a similar expression for E_1 from symmetry. The steady state mean ligation number is then

$$E(\infty) = vN \frac{\kappa(1 + g + \kappa)\mu_0 + (g + (g + \kappa)(g + v\mu_0))\mu_1}{(g + \kappa)(1 + g + \kappa + v(\mu_0 + \mu_1) + v(\kappa\mu_0 + (g + v\mu_0)\mu_1))}$$

which is a rational function of the TF concentration v of degree 2 and is linear in the number of binding sites N. Hence,

$$\eta_H(v) = v \frac{\mathrm{d}\ln(\frac{E(\infty)}{N - E(\infty)})}{\mathrm{d}v} = v \frac{\mathrm{d}}{\mathrm{d}v} \ln(\frac{vR(v)}{1 - vR(v)}),$$

where

$$R(v) = \frac{\kappa(1 + g + \kappa)\mu_0 + (g + (g + \kappa)(g + v\mu_0))\mu_1}{(g + \kappa)(1 + g + \kappa + v(\mu_0 + \mu_1) + v(\kappa\mu_0 + (g + v\mu_0)\mu_1))}.$$

$\eta_H(v)$ does not depend on the number of sites N, and numerical simulations indicate a negative cooperativity in the Hill sense with $\eta_H(v) < 1$. We thus see the drastic effect of allowing conformational changes for arbitrary TF binding configurations.

In the first model, conformational changes occur only when DNA is free of TF, leading to a strong positive cooperativity in the Hill sense. In the second one, no particular restriction is imposed on conformational changes, leading to negative cooperativity in the Hill sense. We finally focus on a model where the chromatin can switch between the ON and OFF states when the DNA is naked, but where it can switch to the accessible state for any configuration of bound TF. The associated set of chemical reactions is again of the form

$$(MX)_k + X \underset{\kappa_{-,y}^{k+1}}{\overset{\kappa_{+,y}^k}{\rightleftharpoons}} (MX)_{k+1},$$

with the constrained switching mechanism

$$\mathcal{O}_0 \underset{0}{\overset{g}{\longleftrightarrow}} \mathcal{O}_1, \text{ when } k > 0, \quad \mathcal{O}_0 \underset{\kappa > 0}{\overset{g}{\longleftrightarrow}} \mathcal{O}_1, \text{ when } k = 0. \tag{7.6}$$

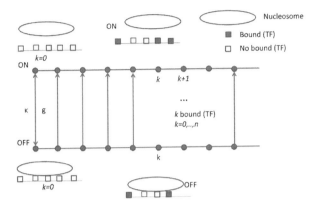

FIGURE 7.10: Transition diagram associated with model (7.6).

One can again use the master equation, and observe that the mean ligation number is obtained by setting $\kappa = 0$ in the preceding model. In this case,

$$\sup_{v} \eta_H(v) = 1,$$

so that the system does not exhibit positive cooperativity in the Hill sense.

Chapter 8

Signalling switches

Section 4.2 focuses on signalling pathways where a linear cascade composed of protein kinases transduces some external signal toward the nucleus. Each kinase can be phosphorylated or dephosphorylated through the action of kinases and phosphatases. More generally, substrate molecules can usually be phosphorylated at multiple sites, with up to 7 sites in prokaryotes, and up to 150 sites in eukaryotes (see, e.g., [172]) leading to a large set of possible phosphoforms. The associated phosphorylation process can be seen as a binding process, and the mathematical tools developed in chapter 5 can be adapted to study signalling switches. We present here some recent mathematical models which aim at explaining the experimentally observed switching-like behaviours of basic signalling modules composed of a kinase, a phosphatase and a substrate, the latter containing N phosphorylation sites where phosphates can bind. Such systems can switch abruptly from an inactive or dephosphorylated state to an active or phosphorylated state when the kinase concentration crosses a critical threshold. More than 30% of the proteins are phosphorylated at possibly multiple sites, and this kind of module is thought to be a fundamental element of cell regulation; see, e.g., [106].

These systems exhibit **ultrasensitivity**: a small change in kinase or phosphatase concentration induces a large change in the proportion of phosphorylated substrate. This switching-like behaviour might be useful when a cell has a binary decision to make, as, for example, differentiation or cell division in the presence of growth factors. Besides ultrasensitivity, pathways containing such modules are useful for inducing **thresholding**, where a small amount of active kinase does not lead to a significant amount of phosphorylated substrate; see, e.g., [91], [76] or [115].

Switches occur generally when the number of binding sites is large; the authors of [76] proved that the dose-response curve associated with fully phosphorylated proteins can lead to poor switches, and [121] showed that ultrasensitivity in phosphorylation-dephosphorylation cycles can occur with litle substrate. The authors of [185] claimed that partially phosphorylated substrate can be as active as the fully phosphorylated one. They hence proposed a model where the substrate is active when more than k_0 sites are bound by phosphates, for some threshold k_0. The next two sections deal with this kind of model, by discussing ordered and unordered phosphorylation processes separately, since it turns out that phosphorylation can occur with some predefined order dictated by biochemical laws, or new sites can be phosphorylated in a random order; see below.

8.1 Ordered phosphorylation

Phosphorylation can be described using enzymatic reactions of the generic form

$$S_i + E \underset{\kappa_-^i}{\overset{\kappa_+^i}{\longleftrightarrow}} SE_i \overset{\kappa_2^i}{\longrightarrow} S_{i+1} + E$$

(see, e.g, [185]), where S_i denotes a substrate molecule having i phosphorylated sites, and where E is the kinase. Notice that this kind of reaction has been considered in section 4.1. Similarly, dephosphorylation is represented by the reactions

$$S_{i+1} + F \underset{l_-^i}{\overset{l_+^i}{\longleftrightarrow}} SF_{i+1} \overset{l_2^i}{\longrightarrow} S_i + F,$$

where F is the phosphatase. Let u be the ratio of the kinase and phosphatase concentrations. In its simplest form, the probability of seeing a substrate having i phosphorylated sites among the $N+1$ possible phosphoforms is, using, for example, the fact that this Markov chain is a birth and death process,

$$\pi(|n| = k) = \frac{\lambda^k u^k}{1 + \lambda u + \cdots + \lambda^N u^N} = \frac{x^k}{x^{N+1} - 1},$$

(see (2.2.3)), for a positive constant $\lambda > 0$, which models the relative phosphorylation efficiency, where we set $x = \lambda u$. Assuming that the substrate is active when the activation threshold is $k_0 = \alpha(N+1)$, for some $0 < \alpha < 1$, the dose-response curve is

$$V_\alpha(x) = \pi(|n| \geq \alpha(N+1)) = \frac{x^{k_0} + x^{k_0+1} + \cdots + x^N}{x^{N+1} - 1} = \frac{x^{N+1} - x^{k_0}}{x^{N+1} - 1}.$$

Let $\bar{x} = x^{N+1}$. The cooperativity index I_p is obtained by looking for quantiles $\bar{x}_p$ such that

$$p = \frac{\bar{x}_p - \bar{x}_p^\alpha}{\bar{x}_p - 1}.$$

When $p = 0.9$, the authors of [185] obtained that

$$I = I_{0.9} \sim 2\alpha(1 - \alpha)(N + 1),$$

which is approximately linear in N for large N. This kind of dose-response curve is steep, and leads to good switches for large N.

8.2 Unordered phosphorylation

In the unordered case, phosphorylation and dephosphorylation steps can occur at any site i, so that one must deal with the full state space $\Lambda = \{n = (n_i)_{1 \leq i \leq N}, \ n_i = 0, 1\}$, giving the possible phosphoforms, of size $|\Lambda| = 2^N$. Recall that $n_i = 1$ means that site i is bound by a phosphate. A transition of the form

$$x = (n_1, \cdots, n_{i-1}, 0, n_{i+1}, \cdots, n_N)$$
$$\longrightarrow y = (n_1, \cdots, n_{i-1}, 1, n_{i+1}, \cdots, n_N)$$

corresponds to the binding of a phosphate at site i through the action of a kinase, and likewise, for dephosphorylation steps

$$x = (n_1, \cdots, n_{i-1}, 1, n_{i+1}, \cdots, n_N)$$
$$\longrightarrow y = (n_1, \cdots, n_{i-1}, 0, n_{i+1}, \cdots, n_N).$$

We furthermore assume that these transitions occur at rates proportional to the concentrations of kinase e and of phosphatase f. In summary, we allow transitions of the form $n \to n + e_i$, when $n_i = 0$, at rate $\kappa_+ e$, and transitions like $n \to n - e_i$, when $n_i = 1$, of rate $\kappa_- f$. The related Markov chain $X(t)$ has a steady state distribution given by the product measure of Bernoulli type

$$\pi(n) = \prod_i \frac{x^{n_i}}{1 + x} = \frac{x^{|n|}}{(1 + x)^N},$$

where we set

$$x = \frac{\kappa_+ e}{\kappa_- f}.$$

Hence,

$$\pi(|n| = i) = \frac{\binom{N}{i} x^i}{(1 + x^N)}.$$

Adopting again an activation threshold of the form $k_0 = \alpha N$, the proportion of active substrate is

$$V_\alpha(x) = \pi(|n| > \alpha N).$$

The above occupation probability is of binomial type, that is, $|n| = S_N$ with

$$S_N = \varepsilon_1 + \cdots + \varepsilon_N,$$

where the random variables ε_i are i.i.d. Bernoulli of success parameter $q = x/(1 + x)$. Large deviation theory shows that

$$\lim_{N \to \infty} \frac{1}{N} \ln(\pi(|n| > \alpha N)) = - \inf_{s > \alpha,\ s \in [0,1]} H_q(s),$$

that is,

$$\pi(|n| > \alpha N) \asymp \exp(-N \inf_{s > \alpha,\ s \in [0,1]} H_q(s)),$$

where $H_q(s)$ is the entropy function

$$H_q(s) = s \ln\left(\frac{s}{q}\right) + (1 - s) \ln\left(\frac{1 - s}{1 - q}\right) \geq 0,$$

which is such that

$$H_q(s) > 0 \text{ when } s \neq q \text{ and } H_q(q) = 0$$

see, e.g,. [45] or [39] and figure 8.1. Hence,

$$\pi(|n| > \alpha N) \asymp \exp(-N H_q(\alpha)),$$

when x is such that $q < \alpha$, that is, when $x < x_c = \alpha/(1 - \alpha)$, with

$$H_q(\alpha) > 0,$$

so that the related probability decreases to zero exponentially fast in N. On the other hand, $\pi(|n| > \alpha N) \sim 1$ when x is larger than the threshold x_c. We then understand why the response curve $V_\alpha(x)$ exhibits switching properties when N is large.

The authors of [185] focused on the 10% and 90% quantiles of the above distribution function. For general p, the cooperativity index I_p is obtained by looking for the quantiles x_p such that

$$V_\alpha(x_p) = p,$$

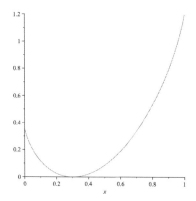

FIGURE 8.1: Plot of $H_q(x)$, for $q = 1/4$.

since $V_\alpha(\infty) = 1$. One thus arrives at

$$
\begin{aligned}
p = V_\alpha(x_p) &= \pi(|n| > k_0) = \pi(S_N > \alpha N) \\
&= \pi(S_N - N\frac{x_p}{1+x_p} > N(\alpha - \frac{x_p}{1+x_p})) \\
&= \pi(\frac{S_N - N\frac{x_p}{1+x_p}}{\sqrt{N\frac{x_p}{1+x_p}\frac{1}{1+x_p}}} > \frac{\sqrt{N}(\alpha - \frac{x_p}{1+x_p})(1+x_p)}{\sqrt{x_p}}).
\end{aligned}
$$

The Central Limit Theorem yields that one must solve the limiting equation

$$
q_\alpha = \frac{\sqrt{N}(\alpha - \frac{x_p}{1+x_p})(1+x_p)}{\sqrt{x_p}},
$$

where q_p is such that

$$
p = \frac{1}{\sqrt{2\pi}} \int_{q_\alpha}^{\infty} e^{-\frac{u^2}{2}} \, du.
$$

Proceeding this way, the authors of [185] obtained that

$$
I = I_{0.9} \sim \frac{\ln(81)}{2q_p} \sqrt{\alpha(1-\alpha)} \sqrt{N},
$$

when N is large, showing that this kind of activation threshold leads to good switches. The probability measure π falls within the context of section 5.9, so that, according to (5.23),

$$
I = I_{0.9} \leq \sup_x \eta_H(x).
$$

Part III

A short course on dynamical systems

Chapter 9

Differential equations, flows and vector fields

We have seen in section 3.1 that for first order linear chemical reaction networks, the mean abundance vector $E(t)$ and the vector containing the second moments $V(t)$ satisfy ordinary differential equations (o.d.e.) that can be deduced from probabilistic arguments; see (3.1) and (3.2). Sections 12.1 and 12.4 will provide a law of large numbers and Gaussian approximations that lead to gaussian processes drifted by nonlinear o.d.e., which are the main actual mathematical tool for handling complex gene regulatory networks. We hence provide a short course on dynamical systems in chapters 9, 10 and 11 for scientists having some knowledge of differential calculus; we will use parts of this material in chapters 12 and 13 when dealing with the linear noise approximation and mass action kinetics.

9.1 Some examples

9.1.1 Malthus and Verhulst equations

One very basic example of ordinary differential equations is the linear one dimensional equation

$$\dot{x} = \frac{dx}{dt} = fx. \tag{9.1}$$

The solution is easily computed to be $x(t) = x(0)e^{tf}$. This can be seen as a naive model of *Malthusian evolution*[1] describing the abundance of some pop-

---

[1] Thomas Robert Malthus, 1766-1834, was a British reverend and economist, most known for his controversial essay published in 1798 entitled *An Essay on the Principle of Population*. In this essay Malthus defends the thesis that the growth of populations is exponential and might have catastrophic consequences if not regulated.

ulation $x(t) \geq 0$. Depending on the sign of the growth rate f, the population either increases to ∞ ($f > 0$) or decreases to zero ($f < 0$) exponentially.

Inspired by the Malthusian evolution model, Pierre François Verhulst[2] proposed around 1840 to model a species evolution with a non-constant growth rate:

$$f(x) = r(1 - \frac{x}{K}).$$

So that

$$\dot{x} = rx(1 - \frac{x}{K}). \tag{9.2}$$

The parameter r is called the intrinsic growth rate and K the *charge capacity*. The sign of $f(x)$ shows that for all $x > 0$,

$$\lim_{t \to \infty} x(t) = K.$$

Exercise 9.1.1 Compute the solutions to (9.2).

9.1.2 Predators-Preys systems: The Lotka-Volterra model

The Lotka-Volterra model, named after Vito Volterra[3] and Alfred Lotka,[4] is a simple model describing two species in interaction. One of the species consists of prey in abundance $x \geq 0$ and the other consists of predators in abundance $y \geq 0$. Suppose that predators eat exclusively prey and that prey have unlimited resources. Suppose furthermore that the growth rates are affine functions: $y \mapsto a - by$ for prey and $x \mapsto dx - c$ for predators, where $a, b, c, d > 0$. These assumptions encompass the qualitative following properties: in the absence of predators (resp. prey) the growth rate of prey (predators) is positive (negative) and decreases (increases) with predators (prey). The associated ordinary differential equation takes the form

$$\begin{cases} \dot{x} = x(a - by), \\ \dot{y} = y(dx - c), \end{cases} \tag{9.3}$$

and is defined on the positive quadrant $E = \mathbb{R}_+^2$. Uniqueness of solutions (Theorem 9.3.1 below) ensures that both E and the boundary faces $\partial_1 E = \{0\} \times \mathbb{R}_+$, $\partial_2 E = \mathbb{R}_+ \times \{0\}$ are invariant. On the boundary $\partial E = \partial_1 E \cup \partial_2 E$ the dynamics is quite simple:

---

[2] Belgium mathematican 1804-1849.
[3] Italian mathematician, 1860-1940.
[4] American mathematician, 1880-1949.

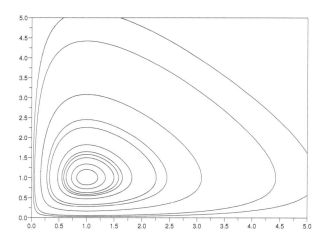

FIGURE 9.1: Phase portrait of equation (9.3).

- The origin $(0,0)$ is a saddle equilibrium.[5]
- On $\partial_2 E$, $\lim_{t\to\infty} x(t) = \infty$ for $x(0) > 0$.
- On $\partial_1 E$, $\lim_{t\to\infty} y(t) = 0$.

In the interior of E there is a unique equilibrium $(x*, y*) = (c/d, a/b)$ and all other trajectories are periodic; see figure 9.1. Indeed, the map $H : \text{int}(E) \to \mathbb{R}$ given by

$$H(x,y) = dx - c\ln(x) + by - a\ln(y)$$

is such that

$$\frac{\mathrm{d}H}{\mathrm{d}t} = -[c/x - d]\dot{x} - [a/y - b]\dot{y} = 0.$$

This implies that H is constant along every trajectory. Furthermore, the Hessian of H at (x,y),

$$\text{Hess}(H) = \begin{pmatrix} c/x^2 & 0 \\ 0 & a/y^2 \end{pmatrix},$$

being positive definite, H is strictly convex. Since $H(x,y) \to \infty$ for $(x,y) \to \partial E$ where $\|(x,y)\| \to \infty$, it follows that, for all $\alpha < H(x^*, y^*)$ the level set $H(x,y) = \alpha$ is a closed curve surrounding (x^*, y^*).

---

[5]See chapter 11 for a formal definition.

Exercise 9.1.2 Show that

$$\frac{1}{T} \int_0^T y(s)\mathrm{d}s = a/b = y^*$$

and

$$\frac{1}{T} \int_0^T x(s)\mathrm{d}s = x^*$$

where $t \mapsto (x(t), y(t))$ is any solution of (9.3), and T is its period.

9.2 Vector fields and differential equations

A **vector field** is a continuous map $F : \mathbb{R}^n \to \mathbb{R}^n$. We consider here the (autonomous) **ordinary differential equation** (o.d.e.)

$$\frac{\mathrm{d}\eta}{\mathrm{d}t} = F(\eta). \tag{9.4}$$

Examples of such o.d.e. are given by (9.1), (9.2) and (9.3). A (local) *solution* to (9.4) is a differentiable map $\eta : I \mapsto \mathbb{R}^n$ defined on a open interval $I \subset \mathbb{R}$ such that $\eta'(t) = F(\eta(t))$ for all $t \in I$. Geometrically $t \mapsto \eta(t)$ is a curve tangent to $F(\eta(t))$ at $\eta(t)$.

If, furthermore, $0 \in I$ and $\eta(0) = x$, η is called the solution to the *Cauchy problem (9.4) with initial condition $x \in \mathbb{R}^n$*.

If $I = \mathbb{R}$, the solution is said to be *global*. A vector field in which all solutions are global is called *globally integrable*.

9.3 Existence and uniqueness theorems

The vector field F is *Lipschitz* if

$$\|F(x) - F(y)\| \leq L\|x - y\|$$

for all $x, y \in \mathbb{R}^n$. L is called the Lipschitz constant of F. It is called *locally Lipschitz* if its restriction to every ball in $\mathbb{R}^n$ is Lipschitz. In particular, by a classical result in differential calculus (the so-called mean value theorem), a C^1 vector field is locally Lipschitz.

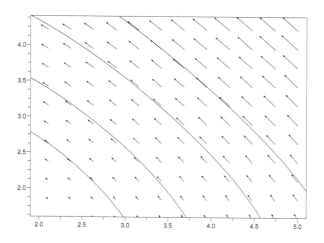

FIGURE 9.2: A vector field and its solution curves.

The following theorem ensures both the existence and the uniqueness of the solution to the Cauchy problem.

Cauchy-Lipschitz Theorem

Theorem 9.3.1 *[Cauchy-Lipchitz Theorem] If F is locally Lipschitz, there exists a solution $\eta :]\alpha, \beta[\to \mathbb{R}^n$ with $-\infty \leq \alpha < 0 < \beta \leq \infty$ to the Cauchy problem (9.4) with initial condition x such that*

(i) *if $\xi : J \to \mathbb{R}^n$ is another solution, then $J \subset]\alpha, \beta[$ and $\eta(t) = \xi(t)$ for all $t \in J$.*

(ii) *If $\beta < \infty$ (respectively $\alpha > -\infty$) $\limsup_{t \to \beta(resp.\alpha)} \|\eta(t)\| = \infty$.*

For a proof of this result one can consult the classical textbook [85] or the new version [86].

The solution η in theorem 9.3.1 is called the *maximal solution* to the Cauchy problem. For simplicity we will just call it *the solution*.

Exercise 9.3.2 Show that the Cauchy problem

$$\begin{cases} \dot{y} = \sqrt{y}, \\ y(0) = 0 \end{cases}$$

admits several solutions.

Exercise 9.3.3 Compute the (maximal) solution to the Cauchy problem

$$\begin{cases} \dot{y} = y^2, \\ y(0) = x > 0. \end{cases}$$

Remark 9.3.4 (Reversibility) If $\eta :]\alpha, \beta[\to \mathbb{R}^n$ is the solution to the Cauchy problem (9.4) with initial conditition x, then the map $\xi :] - \beta, -\alpha[\to \mathbb{R}^n$ defined by $\xi(t) = \eta(-t)$ is the solution to the Cauchy problem

$$\frac{d\xi}{dt} = -F(\xi), \ \xi(0) = x.$$

9.3.1 A global existence criterion

Exercise 9.3.3 shows that global solutions do not always exist. The criterion given in theorem 9.3.6 below provides a sufficent condition which proves to be quite useful. It follows from the classical (and also quite useful) lemma:

Lemma 9.3.5 *(Gronwall's Lemma) Let v be a nonnegative continuous function defined on $[0, T]$. Suppose that for all $0 \le t \le T$,*

$$v(t) \le a \int_0^t v(s)ds + b,$$

for some $a, b \ge 0$. Then, for all $0 \le t \le T$,

$$v(t) \le e^{at}b.$$

PROOF:
   If $a = 0$ there is nothing to prove. If $a > 0$ set $w(t) = \int_0^t v(s)ds + b/a$. Then $\dot{w} = v \le aw$. It follows that $\ln(w(t)) - \ln(w(0)) \le at$. Hence $v(t) \le aw(t) \le e^{at}b$. $\square$

Theorem 9.3.6 *Suppose that F is locally Lipschitz and*

$$\|F(x)\| \le a\|x\| + b,$$

for some constants $a, b \ge 0$. Then F is globally integrable.

PROOF:

Let $\eta :]\alpha, \beta[\mapsto \mathbb{R}^n$ be the maximal solution to the Cauchy problem with initial condition $\eta(0) = x$. For $t \geq 0$, $\|\eta(t)\| \leq \|x\| + \int_0^t [a\|\eta(s)\| + b] ds$, and, by Gronwall's lemma, $\|\eta(t)\| \leq e^{a|t|}(\|x\| + bt)$. Assertion (ii) in Theorem 9.3.1 shows that $\beta = \infty$. Similarly $\alpha = -\infty$, by using remark (9.3.4). $\square$

9.4 Higher order and nonautonomous equations

A *nonautonomous* differential equation takes the form

$$\frac{d\eta}{dt} = G(\eta, t), \qquad (9.5)$$

where $G : \mathbb{R}^n \times \mathbb{R} \to \mathbb{R}^n$. Such an equation can be rewritten as an autonomous system by introducing the new variable $u = t$:

$$\begin{cases} \frac{d\eta}{dt} = G(\eta, u) \\ \frac{du}{dt} = 1. \end{cases}$$

When G is locally Lipschitz, theorem 9.3.1 applies. However, it might be useful to consider (9.5) under a weaker regularity assumption in the t variable. The proof of the following theorem is similar to the proof of theorem 9.3.1.

Theorem 9.4.1 *Let $G : \mathbb{R}^n \times \mathbb{R} \to \mathbb{R}^n$. Suppose that*

(i) *G is measurable in t.*

(ii) *For all $R > 0$ and $T > 0$ there exist constants L and M such that for $\|x\| \leq R, \|y\| \leq R$ and $|t| \leq T$*

$$\|G(x, t) - G(y, t)\| \leq L\|x - y\|$$

and

$$\|G(x, t)\| \leq M.$$

Then, the conclusions of theorem 9.3.1 still hold true if one replaces the autonomous equation (9.4) by the nonautonomous equation (9.5). If, furthermore,

$$G(x, t) \leq a\|x\| + b,$$

then the solutions to (9.5) are global.

A pth order o.d.e. is an equation taking the form

$$\eta^{(p)}(t) = G(\eta(t), \eta'(t), \ldots, \eta^{(p-1)}) \tag{9.6}$$

where $\eta^{(i)}(t) = \dfrac{\mathrm{d}^i \eta}{\mathrm{d}t}$ and G is a continuous function from $\mathbb{R}^n \times \ldots \times \mathbb{R}^n$ into $\mathbb{R}^n$. The change of variable $y_1 = \eta, y_2 = \dot{\eta}, \ldots, y_{p-1} = \eta^{(p-1)}$ transforms the nonautonomous equation (9.5) into an autonomous system

$$\begin{cases} y_1' = y_2, \\ \ldots, \\ y_{p-2}' = y_{p-1}, \\ y_{p-1}' = G(y_0, \ldots, y_{p-1}). \end{cases}$$

Therefore we can (and will) restrict our attention to autonomous systems.

9.5   Flow and phase portrait

We assume here that F verifies the hypotheses of theorem 9.3.1 and (for simplicity) that it is globally integrable. The **flow** induced by F is the mapping

$$\Phi : \mathbb{R} \times \mathbb{R}^n \to \mathbb{R}^n,$$

$$(t, x) \mapsto \Phi_t(x),$$

such that $t \mapsto \Phi_t(x)$ is the solution to the Cauchy problem (9.4) with initial condition x.

Flow properties

Proposition 9.5.1 *(Basic Properties) The mapping Φ is continuous and verifies the following properties:*

(i) $\Phi_0 = \mathrm{Id}$.

(ii) *For all $t, s \in \mathbb{R}$*

$$\Phi_t \circ \Phi_s = \Phi_{t+s}.$$

(iii) *For each $t \in \mathbb{R}$, Φ_t is an homeomorphism, with inverse Φ_{-t}.*

PROOF:

Assertion (i) follows from the definition. To prove (ii), note that $t \mapsto \Phi_{t+s}(x)$ and $t \mapsto \Phi_t(\Phi_s(x))$ are solutions to the same Cauchy problem. (iii) follows from the continuity of Φ combined with (i) and (ii). It remains to prove that Φ is continuous:

a)We first assume that F is bounded, that is, $\|F(x)\| \leq M$ for some $M > 0$. Let $R, T > 0$ be given, and L be the Lipschitz constant of F restricted to $B(0, R + MT)$. For all $x, y \in B(0, R)$, $0 \leq t \leq T$ and $|s| \leq T$,

$$\|\Phi_t(x) - \Phi_s(y)\| \leq \|\Phi_t(y) - \Phi_s(y)) + \|\Phi_t(y) - \Phi_t(x)\|$$

$$\leq M|t - s| + \|\Phi_t(y) - \Phi_t(x)\|.$$

Furthermore

$$\|\Phi_t(y) - \Phi_t(x)\| \leq \|x - y\| + L \int_0^t \|\Phi_s(y) - \Phi_s(x)\| ds.$$

Thus, by Gronwall's Lemma 9.3.5,

$$\|\Phi_t(y) - \Phi_t(x)\| \leq e^{Lt} d(x, y) \leq e^{LT} d(x, y).$$

If now $t < 0$, one applies what precedes to Φ_{-t}. Hence for all $x, y \in B(0, R)$ and $s, t \in [-T, T]$

$$\|\Phi_t(x) - \Phi_s(y)\| \leq M|t - s| + e^{LT}\|x - y\|.$$

This proves that Φ is locally Lipschitz.

b) Suppose now that F is not bounded. Fix $T > 0$ and $x \in \mathbb{R}^n$. By continuity in t of the solutions to 9.4 $t \mapsto \Phi_t(x)$ is continuous and there exists $R > 0$ such that $\Phi_t(x) \in B(0, R)$ for all $|t| \leq T$. Let $f : \mathbb{R}_+ \to [0, 1]$ be a Lipschitz function such that $f(t) = 1$ for $t \leq 2$ and $f(t) = 0$ for $t > 3$. Let $G(y) = f(\|y\|/R)F(y)$ so that G is bounded, locally Lipschitz and coincides with F on $B(0, 2R)$.

The flow Ψ induced by G is continuous. Therefore there exists $\alpha > 0$ such that for all $|t| \leq \alpha \|\Psi_t(x) - \Psi_t(y)\| < R$. In particular $\Psi_t(y) \in B(0, R)$. Since G and F coincide on $B(0, R)$ it follows that Φ and Ψ coincide on $[-T, T] \times B(x, \alpha)$. $\square$

A proof of the next result can be found in classical textbooks, including [79] and [85].

Theorem 9.5.2 *If F is C^k with $k \in \mathbb{N}^* \cup \{\infty\}$, then Φ is C^k. In particular Φ_t is a C^k diffeomorphism.*

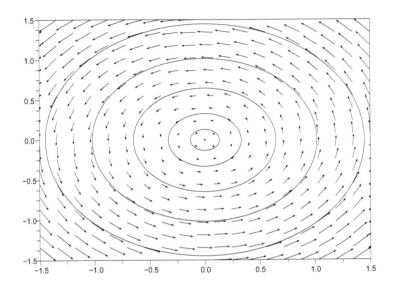

FIGURE 9.3: Phase portrait and vector field corresponding to the system (9.7).

9.5.1 Phase portrait

The state space $\mathbb{R}^n$ is commonly called the **phase space**. A solution $t \mapsto \Phi_t(x)$ can be represented by its graph $\{(t, \Phi_t(x)) : t \in \mathbb{R}^n\}$ in $\mathbb{R} \times \mathbb{R}^n$, or as a parametrised curve in $\mathbb{R}^n$. This latter representation is called the *phase space representation*. The **phase portrait** is the collection of the solution curves in the phase space. We give here a few examples of phase portraits.

Example 9.5.3 The harmonic oscillator

$$\begin{cases} \dot{x} = -\omega y, \\ \dot{y} = \omega x; \end{cases} \tag{9.7}$$

see figure 9.3.

Example 9.5.4 The perturbed harmonic oscillator

$$\begin{cases} \dot{x} = -\omega y + x(1 - (x^2 + y^2)), \\ \dot{y} = \omega x + y(1 - (x^2 + y^2)); \end{cases} \tag{9.8}$$

see figure 9.4.

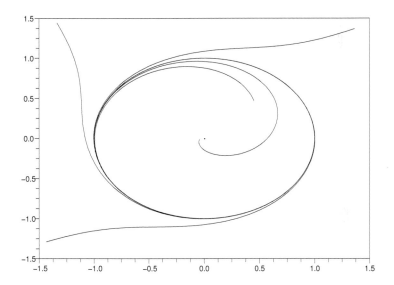

FIGURE 9.4: Phase portrait of (9.8).

9.5.2   The variational equation

We assume F is C^1. Let $DF(x)$ denote the differential of F at point x, which is also known as the **Jacobian matrix** of F at x. Recall that if $F(x) = (F_1(x), \ldots, F_n(x))$, then

$$DF(x) = \left(\frac{\partial F_i}{\partial x_j}(x) \right)_{ij}.$$

The variational equation in x is the nonautonomous differential equation in $M_n(\mathbb{R})$ (the space of $n \times n$ real matrices)

$$\frac{\mathrm{d}M(t)}{\mathrm{d}t} = DF(\Phi_t(x))M(t). \tag{9.9}$$

Theorem 9.4.1 shows that for every initial condition $M(0) = M \in M_n(\mathbb{R})$ (9.9) admits a unique solution.

Proposition 9.5.5 *The differential of Φ_t in x, $D\Phi_t(x)$ is the solution to the variational equation (9.9) with initial condition $M(0) = \mathrm{Id}$.*

PROOF:

$$\Phi_t(x) = x + \int_0^t F(\Phi_s(x))\mathrm{d}s.$$

Since $x, s \rightarrow F(\Phi_s(x))$ is C^1 one can differentiate under the integral. Hence

$$D\Phi_t(x) = \mathrm{Id} + \int_0^t DF(\Phi_s(x))D\Phi_s(x)\mathrm{d}s.$$

□

Exercise 9.5.6 Deduce from proposition (9.5.5) that $D\Phi_t(x)F(x) = F(\Phi_t(x))$.

9.5.2.1   Liouville formula

The *divergence* of F at point x is the trace of $DF(x)$:

$$\mathrm{div}(F)(x) = \mathrm{Tr}(DF(x)) = \sum_{i=1}^n \frac{\partial F_i}{\partial x_i}(x).$$

Proposition 9.5.7 *(Liouville formula) The determinant of $D\Phi_t(x)$ is given as*

$$\det(D\Phi_t(x)) = \exp\left(\int_0^t \mathrm{div}(F)(\Phi_s(x))\mathrm{d}s \right).$$

This formula allows the computation (or at least the estimation) of the temporal evolution of a volume of initial conditions in the phase space. Indeed, if $A \subset \mathbb{R}^n$ is a (measurable) set having volume $\lambda(A)$, then, by the change of variables formula,

$$\lambda(\Phi_t(A)) = \int_A |\det(\mathrm{D}\Phi_t(x))| \mathrm{d}x.$$

Then

$$\lambda(\Phi_t(A)) = \int_A \exp\left(\int_0^t \mathrm{div}(F)(\Phi_s(x))\mathrm{d}s\right)\mathrm{d}x. \tag{9.10}$$

In particular

Corollary 9.5.8 *If F has zero divergence, Φ_t preserves the volume in the phase space.*

Example 9.5.9 Let $F : \mathbb{R}^2 \to \mathbb{R}^2$ be a C^1 vector field. It is called *Hamiltonian* if

$$F(x, y) = \begin{cases} \frac{\partial H}{\partial y}(x, y), \\ -\frac{\partial H}{\partial x}(x, y), \end{cases}$$

for some C^2 function $H : \mathbb{R}^2 \to \mathbb{R}$. The divergence of such an F is nul, hence the flow of F preserves the surfaces in the plane. Note also that H is constant along trajectories since

$$\frac{\mathrm{d}H}{\mathrm{d}t} = \frac{\partial H}{\partial x}(x, y) + \dot{x}\frac{\partial H}{\partial y}(x, y)\dot{y} = 0.$$

Exercise 9.5.10 Show that, conversely, every C^2 vector field $F : \mathbb{R}^2 \mapsto \mathbb{R}^2$ having zero divergence is hamiltonian.

The proof of Liouville's formula follows from the variational equation and the next lemma:

Lemma 9.5.11 *Let $A : \mathbb{R} \to M_n(\mathbb{R})$ be a continuous map, $a(t) = \mathrm{Tr}(A(t))$, and let $M : \mathbb{R} \to M_n(\mathbb{R})$ be the solution to the Cauchy problem*

$$\frac{\mathrm{d}M}{\mathrm{d}t} = A(t)M,$$

with initial condition $M(0) = M_0$. Then $\det(M(t))$ is the solution to the differential equation $\dot{y} = a(t)y$ with initial condition $y(0) = \det(M_0)$. Hence

$$\det(M(t)) = \det(M_0)\exp\left(\int_0^t a(s)\mathrm{d}s\right).$$

PROOF:

Fix $t \in \mathbb{R}$. Then $M(t+s) = M(t)+M'(t)s+o(s) = M(t)(\mathrm{Id}+sA(t)M(t)+o(s))$. The determinant being a polynomial (hence C^1) of the entries $y(t + s) = y(t)\det(\mathrm{Id} + sA(t)) + o(s)$ where $y(t) = \det(M(t))$. Furthermore $\det(\mathrm{Id} + sA(t)) = 1 + s\mathrm{Tr}(A(t)) + O(s^2)$. This can be deduced, for example, from the formula $\det(A) = \sum_{\sigma \in S_n} \varepsilon(\sigma) \prod_i A_{i,\sigma i}$. Finally

$$\lim_{s \to 0} \frac{y(t + s) - y(t)}{s} = y(t)\mathrm{Tr}(A(t)).$$

$\square$

Chapter 10

Equilibria, periodic orbits and limit cycles

Throughout this chapter, F is a sufficiently regular and globally integrable vector field, and $\Phi = \{\Phi_t\}$ denotes the associated flow.

10.1 Equilibria, periodic orbits and invariant sets

Let $x \in \mathbb{R}^n$. The **trajectory** or the **orbit** of x is the set

$$\gamma(x) = \{\Phi_t(x) : t \in \mathbb{R}\}.$$

The *positive trajectory* is the set

$$\gamma^+(x) = \{\Phi_t(x) : t \geq 0\}.$$

The negative trajectory $\gamma^-(x)$ is similarly defined for $t \leq 0$. An **equilibrium** (or stationary point) is a point $x \in \mathbb{R}^n$ such that

$$F(x) = 0,$$

or, equivalently,

$$\Phi_t(x) = x,$$

for all $t \in \mathbb{R}$. A **periodic point** is a point x such that

(i) x is not an equilibrium, and

(ii)

$$\Phi_T(x) = x,$$

for some $T > 0$.

If x is periodic, the *period* of x is the smallest $T > 0$ such that $\Phi_T(x) = x$. If x is periodic with period T, the orbit of x is a *periodic trajectory* having period T.

A set A is called **positively (respectively negatively) invariant** if $\Phi_t(A) \subset A$ for all $t \geq 0$ (resp. $t \leq 0$).

It is called **invariant** if it is both positively and negatively invariant. Note that if A is invariant, $\Phi_t(A) = A$ for all $t \in \mathbb{R}$.

10.2   Alpha and omega limit sets

A large part of the modern theory of dynamical systems is devoted to the qualitative description of the asymptotic behaviour of trajectories. The *alpha and omega limit* sets are natural objects to describe such behaviours.

The omega limit set of x, denoted $\omega(x)$, is the set of points $p \in \mathbb{R}^n$ such that

$$p = \lim_{n \to \infty} \Phi_{t_n}(x),$$

for some sequence $t_n \to \infty$. In other words, $\omega(x)$ is the set of limit points of $t \mapsto \Phi_t(x)$. **The alpha limit set**, denoted $\alpha(x)$, is the omega limit set of x for the reversed flow $\{\Phi_{-t}\}$.

Properties of limit sets

Proposition 10.2.1 *Suppose that* $\gamma^+(x) = \{\Phi_t(x) : t \geq 0\}$ *is bounded. Then*

(i) $\omega(x)$ *is a non-empty compact connected set invariant under* Φ,

(ii)
$$\overline{\gamma^+}(x) = \gamma^+(x) \cup \omega(x),$$

(iii)
$$\lim_{t \to \infty} \text{dist}(\Phi_t(x), \omega(x)) = 0.$$

PROOF:
    If $\gamma^+(x)$ is bounded, its closure is compact and $\omega(x)$ is bounded and nonempty.

Let $p_n \in \omega(x)$ with $p_n \to p$. Then for all n there exists $t_n > n$ such that $\|\Phi_{t_n}(x) - p_n\| \le 1/n$. Thus $\Phi_{t_n}(x) \to p$ and $p \in \omega(x)$. This proves that $\omega(x)$ is compact.

Invariance is obvious since if $\Phi_{t_n}(x) \to p$ then for all $s \in \mathbb{R}$ $\Phi_{t_n+s}(x) = \Phi_s(\Phi_{t_n}(x)) \to \Phi_s(p)$.

To prove the connectivity, suppose that $\omega(x) \subset U \cup V$ where U and V are two disjoint open sets. If $\omega(x)$ meets U and V there exist sequences (t_n) and (r_n) with $r_n > t_n \to \infty$ such that $\Phi_{t_n}(x) \in U$ and $\Phi_{r_n}(x) \in V$. In particular there exists $s_n \in]t_n, r_n[$ such that $\Phi_{s_n}(x) \in \mathbb{R}^n \setminus (U \cup V)$. By compactness one can assume that $\Phi_{s_n}(x) \to q \in \mathbb{R}^n \setminus (U \cup V)$. This proves that $\omega(x)$ meets $\mathbb{R}^n \setminus (U \cup V)$. A contradiction. Assertions (ii) and (iii) easily follow from compactness. $\square$

Remark 10.2.2 If x is an equilibrium or a periodic point then $\gamma(x) = \omega(x)$.

Exercise 10.2.3 Show that in dimension 1, the limit set of a bounded trajectory is an equilibrium.

Exercise 10.2.4 Let F and G be two vector fields locally Lipschitz in $\mathbb{R}^n$. Suppose

$$G(x) = f(x)F(x),$$

where f is a real valued bounded nonnegative function such that

$$f(x) = 0 \Rightarrow F(x) = 0.$$

Let $\gamma_F(x)$ (respectively $\gamma_G(x)$) be the trajectory based at x for the o.d.e. induced by F (respectively G) and $\omega_F(x)$ (respectively $\omega_G(x)$) be its omega limit set. Prove that $\gamma_F(x) = \gamma_G(x)$ and $\omega_F(x) = \omega_G(x)$.

10.2.1 Limit cycles

A periodic orbit γ which is the (omega or alpha) limit set of a point $x \notin \gamma$ is called a **limit cycle**. In example 9.5.4, the unit circle is the omega limit set of every point distinct from the origin.

10.2.2 Heteroclinic cycle: The May and Leonard example

Let $p_1, \ldots, p_n$ be equilibria and $\gamma_1, \gamma_2, \ldots, \gamma_n$ some orbits such that $p_i = \alpha(\gamma_i)$ and $p_{i+1} = \omega(\gamma_i)$ for $i = 1, \ldots, n$ with the convention $p_{n+1} = p_1$. The set $\Gamma = \{p_1\} \cup \gamma_1 \cup \ldots \{p_n\} \cup \gamma_n$ is called an **heteroclinic** and we write

$$\Gamma : p_1 \hookrightarrow p_2 \hookrightarrow \ldots \hookrightarrow p_n \hookrightarrow p_1.$$

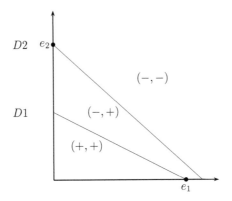

FIGURE 10.1: Signs of $(\dot{x}, \dot{y})$ and isoclines of (10.2).

When $n = 1$, γ_1 is called an **homoclinic** orbit.

The following example is due to May and Leonard [122]. It is a Lotka-Volterra type system involving three species. The dynamics takes place in $E = \mathbb{R}^3_+$ and is given by the system

$$
\begin{cases}
\dot{x} = x(1 - x - \alpha y - \beta z), \\
\dot{y} = y(1 - \beta x - y - \alpha z), \\
\dot{z} = z(1 - \alpha x - \beta y - z),
\end{cases}
\tag{10.1}
$$

where $0 < \beta < 1 < \alpha$. In the absence of species 2 and 3 (that is, when $y = z = 0$) species 1 follows a Verhulst type dynamics (see section 9.1.1). In the absence of species 3 (that is, when $z = 0$) the dynamics in (x, y) on $\partial_3 E = \mathbb{R}^2_+ \times \{0\}$ is given by the system

$$
\begin{cases}
\dot{x} = x(1 - x - \alpha y), \\
\dot{y} = y(1 - \beta x - y);
\end{cases}
\tag{10.2}
$$

see figure 10.2. The lines $D1 : 1 - x - \alpha y = 0$ and $D2 : 1 - \beta x - y = 0$ have empty intersection in $\partial_3 E$ and divide the plane $\partial_3 E$ in three domains in which the signs of $\dot{x}$ and $\dot{y}$ are constant (see figure 10.1).

It then follows that for all $x(0) > 0$, $y(0) > 0$ and $z(0) = 0$ $(x(t), y(t), z(t)) = (x(t), y(t), 0)$ converge toward $e_2 = (0, 1, 0)$. In other words

In the absence of 3, species 2 dominates species 1.

And by symmetry,

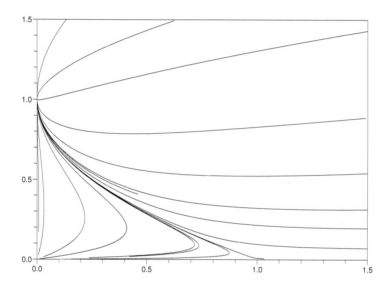

FIGURE 10.2: Phase portrait of (10.2) for $\alpha = 3$ and $\beta = 0.8$.

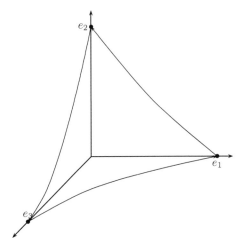

FIGURE 10.3: The heteroclinic cycle $\Gamma : e_1 \hookrightarrow e_2 \hookrightarrow e_3 \hookrightarrow e_1$.

In the absence of 1, 3 *dominates* 2 *and in the absence of* 2, 1 *dominates* 3.

Such a "cyclic competition" reminds one of the Condorcet paradox or the zero sum game "Rock Scissors Paper." The Rock breaks the Scissors which cuts the Paper, which covers the Rock.

   The diagonal $\Delta = \{(x, y, z) \in E : x = y = z\}$ is an invariant set on which the dynamics can be rewritten as

$$\dot{u} = u(1 - u(1 + \alpha + \beta)).$$

The point

$$\left(\frac{1}{1 + \alpha + \beta}, \frac{1}{1 + \alpha + \beta}, \frac{1}{1 + \alpha + \beta} \right)$$

is an equilibrium attracting all the trajectories in Δ.

   A rigorous proof of the following proposition can be found in [87], chapter 5.

Proposition 10.2.5 *There exists an heteroclinic orbit* $\Gamma : e_1 \hookrightarrow e_2 \hookrightarrow e_3 \hookrightarrow e_1$.

   If $\alpha + \beta < 2$, Γ *is the limit set of every point in* $\mathsf{int}(E) \setminus \Delta$.

10.3   The Poincaré-Bendixson theorem

The following celebrated Poincaré-Bendixson theorem characterizes the limit sets in the plane under the generic assumption that equilibria are isolated. It was first stated by the famous French mathematician Henri Poincaré in 1881, and the proof was later completed by Ivar Bendixson in 1901.

Poincaré-Bendixson Theorem

Theorem 10.3.1 *Let $F : \mathbb{R}^2 \to \mathbb{R}^2$ be a C^1 vector field and Φ the associated flow. Let $\omega(x)$ be an nonempty compact omega limit set (i.e. $\gamma^+(x)$ is bounded). Assume that F restricted to $\omega(x)$ has finitely many zeros. $\omega(x)$ is either*

(i) *an equilibrium,*

(ii) *an heteroclinic cycle,*

(iii) *a periodic orbit.*

The next results are easy, but often useful, consequences of this latter theorem.

Corollary 10.3.2 *Under the assumptions of theorem 10.3.1, if $\omega(x)$ contains no equilibrium, it is a periodic orbit.*

Corollary 10.3.3 *If K is a compact positively invariant set, either it contains an equilibrium or a periodic orbit*

The proof of theorem 10.3.1 can be found in [79].

10.4   Chaos

In dimension 1 every alpha or omega limit set (for a bounded trajectory) consists of equilibria (see exercice 10.2.3). In dimension 2 (see section 10.3), it may also be a periodic orbit or an heteroclinic cycle. In larger dimensions

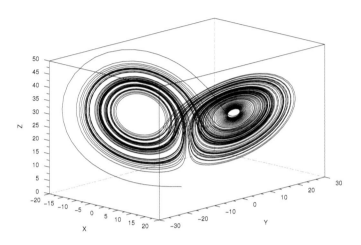

FIGURE 10.4: The Lorenz Attractor.

the structure of limit sets is much richer. It is easy to construct toral limit sets (see exercise (10.6.2)), and there are dynamics which exhibit *chaotic behaviours*. Deterministic chaos in small dimensions is a relatively new discovery. It goes back to 1963 with the discovery by Edward Norton Lorenz[1] of what is now known as the *Lorenz Attractor*. Before Lorenz we believed that turbulent behaviours required a large number of degrees of freedom. Since the work of Lorenz we know that three dimensional differential equations can produce "deterministic chaos." Lorenz wanted to explain with a simple model certain climate phenomena. With this purpose, he considered fluid in a two dimensional box heated from above and cooled down from below. Drastic simplifications of fluid mechanics equations led him to consider the following system:

$$\begin{cases} \dot{x} = \sigma(y - x), \\ \dot{y} = \rho x - y - xz, \\ \dot{z} = xy - \beta z. \end{cases} \qquad (10.3)$$

The x variable is proportional to the convection intensity, y and z are related to temperature variations, σ and ρ are the Prandtl constant and the Rayleigh number. Finally β is a dimensional parameter.

For $\sigma = 10, \beta = 8/3$ and $\rho = 28$, Lorenz observed experimentally (using

---

[1] American meteorologist, professor at MIT, 1917-2008.

a Royal McBee LGP-30) that all but equilibria trajectories converge toward a strange attractor $\mathcal{L}$ consisting of two kinds of lobes (see figure 10.4), and seem to jump from one to another in an erratic fashion. Furthermore, trajectories based at arbitrary close initial conditions eventually split up. Such a property is now known as the *sensitivity to initial conditions* or *butterfly effect* characteristic of chaotic systems.

While the simple form of (10.3) easily allows its numerical investigation, the formal proof of chaotic behaviour is complicated and actually not yet completely achieved. Certain approximations of the Lorenz system, called *geometrical models*, were studied by Guckenheimer and Williams in 1979 (see, e.g., chapter 14 in [86]). It was recently proved by Tucker in 1999 [174] that for certain parameter values the real Lorenz model is equivalent to these geometrical models. For these *geometrical models* the set $\mathcal{L}$ has the following properties:

(i) It is an attractor (see section 10.6);

(ii) Topological transitivity: there exists a dense orbit in $\mathcal{L}$;

(iv) Periodic orbit are dense in $\mathcal{L}$;

(v) The system is *sensitive to initial conditions*: there exists $a > 0$ such that
$$\forall \varepsilon > 0, \ \forall x \in A \ : \sup_{t \geq 0, \, y \in B(x, \varepsilon)} \| \Phi_t(x) - \Phi_t(y) \| \geq a.$$

These properties define *a strange attractor*.

10.4.1 Lotka-Volterra and chaos

The Lotka-Volterra system with two prey and one predator given by

$$\begin{cases} \dot{x} = x(1 - x - y - 10z), \\ \dot{y} = y(1 - 1.5x - y - z), \\ \dot{z} = z(-1 + 5x + 0.5y - 0.01z) \end{cases} \tag{10.4}$$

has been proposed by Gilpin [68] (see also [87] exercise 16.2.9)). Numerical simulations seem to indicate the presence of a strange attractor; see figure 10.5.

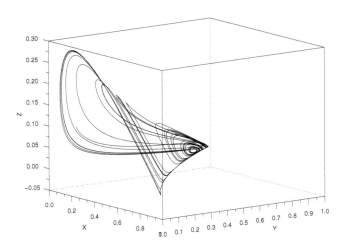

FIGURE 10.5: The attractor of the system (10.4).

10.5   Lyapunov functions

A **Lyapunov function** is a continuous map $V : \mathbb{R}^n \to \mathbb{R}$ that is decreasing along trajectories: for all $x \in \mathbb{R}^n$ and $t \geq 0$,

$$V(\Phi_t(x)) \leq V(x).$$

If V is differentiable, this amounts to saying that

$$\frac{d}{dt}V(\Phi_t(x))_{t=0} = \langle \nabla V(x), F(x) \rangle \leq 0$$

for all x.

Theorem 10.5.1 *Let V be a Lyapunov function and $x \in \mathbb{R}^n$ such that $\gamma^+(x)$ (respectively $\gamma^-(x)$) is bounded. Then V is constant on $\omega(x)$ (respectively $\alpha(x)$).*

PROOF:

Suppose that V is nonconstant on $\omega(x)$. Then there exist $p, q \in \omega(x)$ with $V(q) > V(p)$. By continuity of V there exist O_p neighbourhoods of p and O_q neighbourhoods of q such that $V(w) > V(u)$ for all $u \in O_p, w \in O_q$. On the other hand, there are $s_1, s_2 > 0$ such that $u = \Phi_{s_1}(x) \in O_p$ and

$w = \Phi_{s_1+s_2}(x) = \Phi_{s_2}(u) \in O_q$. This is in contradiction to the monotonicity of $t \mapsto V(\Phi_t(x))$. $\square$

The following corollary is sometimes called the **LaSalle invariance principle**.

Corollary 10.5.2 *Let V be a differentiable Lyapunov function and*

$$\Lambda = \{x \in \mathbb{R}^n \; : \; \langle \nabla V(x), F(x) \rangle = 0\}.$$

Then, for all $x \in \mathbb{R}^n$ such that $\gamma^+(x)$ (respectively $\gamma^-(x)$) is bounded, $\omega(x)$ (respectively $\alpha(x)$) is a compact connected invariant subset of Λ.

PROOF:

For all $p \in \omega(x)$ and $t \in \mathbb{R}$ $V(\Phi_t(p)) = V(p)$ because $\omega(x)$ is invariant and V is constant on $\omega(x)$. Hence, by taking the derivative, $\langle \nabla V(p), F(p) \rangle = 0$. $\square$

A Lyapunov function V is called a *strict Lyapunov* function if the set Λ in corollary 10.5.2 coincides with the equilibria (i.e. the zeros of F).

Corollary 10.5.3 *Assume that there exists a strict Lyapunov function for F and that the equilibria of F are isolated. Then every bounded trajectory converges toward an equilibrium.*

Example 10.5.4 A gradient vector field is a vector field taking the form

$$F(x) = -\nabla V(x).$$

For such a field, V is a strict Lyapunov function.

10.6   Attractors

A set A is called an **attractor** provided

(i) A is compact and invariant,

(ii) there exists a neighbourhood U of A such that

$$\lim_{t \to \infty} \text{dist}(\Phi_t(x), A) = 0$$

uniformly in $x \in U$. That is: For all $\varepsilon > 0$ there exists $T > 0$ such that for all $x \in U$ and $t \geq T$ $\text{dist}(\Phi_t(x), A) \leq \varepsilon$.

The **basin of attraction** of attractor A is the open set

$$B(A) = \{x \in \mathbb{R}^n; \omega(x) \in A\} = \cup_{t \geq 0} \Phi_{-t}(U).$$

If $B(A) = \mathbb{R}^n$ A is called a *global* attractor and F is said to be *dissipative*.

Example 10.6.1 In example 9.5.4, the unit disk D and the unit circle ∂D are both attractors. The basin of D is $\mathbb{R}^2$ and the basin of ∂D is $\mathbb{R}^2 \setminus \{0, 0\}$.

Observe that with such a definition, an attractor may contain other attractors. An attractor A will be called *minimal* or *topologically transitive* provided it admits a dense orbit.

Exercise 10.6.2 Let $F_\omega : \mathbb{R}^2 \mapsto \mathbb{R}^2$ be the vector field given by (9.8). Consider the differential equation in $\mathbb{R}^4$

$$\begin{cases} (\dot{x}, \dot{y}) = F_1(x, y), \\ (\dot{u}, \dot{v}) = F_\omega(u, v). \end{cases}$$

Show that the torus $S^1 \times S^1$ (where S^1 is the unit disk in $\mathbb{R}^2$) is an attractor. Determine its basin. For which value of ω is this attractor minimal ? Discuss the nature of omega limit sets in terms of ω.

Exercise 10.6.3 Consider the differential equation in $\mathbb{R}^2$ given (in polar coordinates) by

$$\begin{cases} \dot{\rho} = \rho(1 - \rho), \\ \dot{\theta} = \sin(\theta/2)^2. \end{cases}$$

Sketch the phase portrait. Determine attractors and limit sets.

10.7   Stability in autonomous systems

Let $a \in \mathbb{R}^n$ be an equilibrium point of the autonomous system

$$\frac{d\eta}{dt} = F(\eta),$$

with $F(a) = 0$. Let $B(a, R)$ be the ball of radius $R > 0$ of center a,

$$B(a, R) = \{x \in \mathbb{R}^n; \ ||x - a|| < R\},$$

where $||x||$ is the norm of x. Let $S(a, R)$ be the sphere

$$S(a, R) = \{x \in \mathbb{R}^n; \ ||x - a|| = R\}.$$

Suppose that the above o.d.e. is well defined in $B(a, A)$ for some positive $A > 0$; in particular, we assume that the partial derivatives of F all exist and are continuous in this domain.

- We say that a is **stable** whenever for each $R < A$ there is an $r \leq R$ such that if an orbit γ^+ initiates at x_0 of $B(a, r)$ then it remains in $B(a, R)$, and never reaches the boundary $S(a, R)$ of $B(a, R)$.

- a is an **asymptotically stable equilibrium** whenever it is stable and in addition every orbit γ^+ starting inside some $B(a, R_0)$, $R_0 > 0$, converges to a as time increases.

- a is an **unstable** equilibrium whenever for some R and any r, there is always a point $x \in B(a, r)$ such that $\gamma^+(x)$ reaches the boundary $S(a, R)$.

10.8 Application to Lotka-Volterra equations

10.8.1 Lotka-Volterra with limited growth

In the Lotka-Volterra prey-predator model introduced in chapter 9, the prey has unlimited resources. To obtain a more realistic model one can add a competition term among the prey, and similarly among the predators. This leads to the following system:

$$\begin{cases} \dot{x} = x(a - by - \lambda x), \\ \dot{y} = y(dx - c - \mu y), \end{cases} \tag{10.5}$$

where $a, b, c, d, \lambda > 0$ and $\mu \geq 0$.

The dynamics on the boundary of the state space $E = \mathbb{R}_+^2$ is as follows:
- The origin $(0, 0)$ is an equilibrium.
- On $\partial_1 E = \{0\} \times \mathbb{R}_+, y(t) \to 0$.
- On $\partial_2 E = \mathbb{R}_+ \times \{0\}, x(t) \to a/\lambda$ for $x(0) > 0$.

Let $A = (a/\lambda, 0)$. There are two possibilities; see figures 10.6 and 10.6:

(i) there is no equilibrium in $\text{int}(E)$. In this case all the trajectories based in $\text{int}(E)$ converge toward A,

(ii) there exists an equilibrium B in $\text{int}(E)$ and, in this case, all the trajectories based in $\text{int}(E)$ converge toward B.

To prove this result, first notice that the compact set

$$\{(x,y) : 0 \le x \le a/\lambda, 0 \le y \le \mu a/\lambda - c\}$$

is positively invariant and attracts all the trajectories.

- If the lines $D1 : a = by + \lambda x$ and $D2 : c = dx - \mu y$ do not intersect in $\text{int}(E)$, they separate $\text{int}(E)$ into three sets and by looking at the vector field in each of these sets one easily sees that the trajectories converge toward A. The reasoning is similar to what has been done with the May and Leonard model (equation (10.2)) and the proof is left to the reader.

- If $D1$ and $D2$ do not intersect in $\text{int}(E)$, they must intersect in a unique point $B = (x^*, y^*)$. The function $V : \text{int}(E) \to \mathbb{R}$ defined as

$$V(x,y) = -d(x^* \ln(x) - x) - b(y^* \ln(y) - y),$$

is a strict Lyapunov function. Indeed, using the fact that $a = by^* + \lambda x^*$ and $c = dx^* - \mu y^*$ one obtains

$$\dot{V}(x,y) = -[d(x^* - x)(by^* + \lambda x^* - by - \lambda x) + b(y^* - y)(-dx^* + \mu y^* + dx - fy)]$$

$$= -d\lambda(x^* - x)^2 - b\mu(y^* - y)^2 \le 0$$

Since, furthermore, $V(x,y) \to \infty$ when $(x,y) \to \partial E$ it follows that $\omega(x,y) \cap \partial E = \emptyset$ for all $(x,y) \in \text{Int}(E)$. Finally, thanks to proposition 10.5.2, $\omega(x,y) = B$.

10.8.2   Lotka-Volterra in dimension n

A Lotka-Volterra system in dimension n can be written in the general form

$$\dot{x}_i = x_i(b_i - \sum_j a_{ij} x_j). \tag{10.6}$$

The term b_i is the intrinsic growth rate of species i, and a_{ij} is the interaction coefficient between species j and i. The matrix $A = (a_{ij})$ is called the *interaction matrix*. The state space is the positive orthant $E = \mathbb{R}^n_+$.

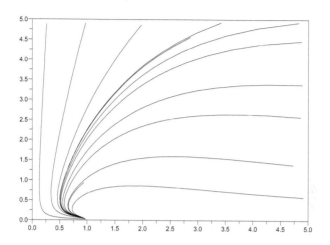

FIGURE 10.6: Phase portrait of equation (10.5), case (*i*).

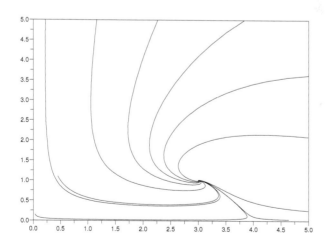

FIGURE 10.7: Phase portrait of equation (10.5), case (*ii*).

Symmetric interactions

Suppose that A is symmetric. Then the function

$$V(x) = \sum_i b_i x_i - \frac{1}{2} \sum_{i,j} a_{ij} x_i x_j$$

is a strict Lyapunov function for (10.6). Indeed,

$$\frac{\partial V}{\partial x_i} = b_i - \sum_j a_{ij} x_j,$$

so that

$$\dot{V} = \sum_i x_i (b_i - \sum_j a_{ij} x_j)^2.$$

Corollary 10.5.2 then shows that

Proposition 10.8.1 *If A is symmetric, the omega limit set of every bounded solution to (10.6) consists of equilibria.*

Exercise 10.8.2 Prove that there "generically" are at most finitely many equilibria for (10.6). Deduce that, generically, every trajectory in a competitive Lotka-Volterra with symmetric interactions (i.e. $a_{ij} = a_{ji} > 0$) converges toward an equilibrium.

Persistence

An ecological system describing species interactions is called *persistent* if all the species coexist. The dynamics (10.6) will then be called persistent if for every bounded trajectory $\gamma^+(x)$

$$x \in \text{int}(E) \Rightarrow \omega(x) \subset \text{int}(E).$$

Proposition 10.8.3 *If (10.6) has no equilibrium in $\text{Int}(E)$ then (10.6) is not persistent.*

PROOF:

The set $C = A(\text{Int}(E))$ is convex. Thus, if $b \notin C$ there exists an hyperplane through b which doesn't meet C. There exists a unit vector c orthogonal to this hyperplan and such that for all $x \in \text{Int}(E)$ $\langle Ax - b, c \rangle > 0$. Let $V : \text{Int}(E) \to \mathbb{R}$ be the map defined by

$$V(x) = \sum_i c_i \ln(x_i).$$

Then $\dot{V} = -\langle Ax - b, c \rangle < 0$. By theorem 10.5.1 no compact limit set can be contained in $\text{Int}(E)$. $\square$

Chapter 11

Linearisation

11.1 Linear differential equations

Let $M_n(\mathbb{R})$ denote the space of $n \times n$ matrices with real entries. Given $A \in M_n(\mathbb{R})$, we let

$$\|A\| = \sup_{x \neq 0} \frac{\|Ax\|}{\|x\|}$$

denote its *operator norm*. Recall that the *exponential of A*, denoted by e^A, is the matrix

$$e^A = \sum_{k \geq 0} \frac{A^k}{k!},$$

which is well defined because $\|A^k\| \leq \|A\|^k$ so that the power series with general term $\frac{A^k}{k!}$ converges in $M_n(\mathbb{R})$.

Exercise 11.1.1 Show that if A and B commute then $e^{A+B} = e^A e^B$. Show that $e^{-A} = (e^A)^{-1}$.

One now considers the linear system

$$\frac{\mathrm{d}x}{\mathrm{d}t} = Ax. \tag{11.1}$$

According to theorem 9.3.6, this system is globally integrable and defines a flow $\Phi^A : \mathbb{R}^n \times \mathbb{R} \to \mathbb{R}^n$.

Proposition 11.1.2 *For all $x \in \mathbb{R}^n, t \in \mathbb{R}$,*

$$\Phi_t^A(x) = e^{tA}x.$$

PROOF:

Let $h(t) = e^{tA}x$. One has $h(0) = x$ and $h(t) = \sum_k \frac{t^k A^k}{k!}x = x + tAx + o(t^2)$. Hence $h'(0) = Ax$. Since $h(t+s) = e^{tA}h(s)$ it follows that $h'(t) = e^{tA}h'(0) = e^{tA}Ax = Ae^{tA}x = Ah(t)$. $\square$

The linear nature of Φ^A allows us to describe the asymptotic behaviour of the trajectories $t \mapsto \Phi_t^A(x)$ in terms of the eigenvalues of A. If λ is a real eigenvalue of A and u is the associated eigenvector (i.e. $Au = \lambda u$) then

$$e^{tA}u = e^{\lambda t}u.$$

This follows from the (easily checked fact) that $t \to e^{t\lambda}u$ is the solution to the Cauchy problem 11.1 with initial condition u. If A is diagonalizable, there exists a basis consisting of eigenvectors and the dynamics is given by the dynamics in each eigendirection.

More generally, let $\Lambda(A) \subset \mathbb{C}$ be the set of eigenvalues of A and for each $\lambda \in \Lambda(A)$, let $\alpha(\lambda)$ denote its multiplicity. Although A has real entries it is useful to see A as an operator acting on $\mathbb{C}^n$. The *characteristic space* associated with λ is the vector subspace of $\mathbb{C}^n$

$$G_\lambda = \mathrm{Ker}\left((A - \lambda I)^{\alpha(\lambda)}\right) = \{z \in \mathbb{C}^n : (A - \lambda I)^{\alpha(\lambda)}z = 0\}.$$

Let E_λ be the real vector space defined as

$$E_\lambda = G_\lambda \cap \mathbb{R}^n, \text{ if } \lambda \in \mathbb{R},$$

and

$$E_\lambda = (G_\lambda \bigoplus G_{\bar{\lambda}}) \cap \mathbb{R}^n, \text{ if } \lambda \in \mathbb{C} \setminus \mathbb{R}.$$

Proposition 11.1.3 (i) *Each E_λ is invariant under A and e^{tA};*

(ii) *$\mathbb{R}^n$ is the direct sum of the spaces E_λ;*

(iii) *There exists $C_\lambda > 0$ such that for all $x \in E_\lambda$ and $t \in \mathbb{R}$*

$$\frac{1}{C_\lambda(1 + |t|^k)}e^{t\Re(\lambda)}\|x\| \leq \|e^{tA}x\| \leq C_\lambda(1 + |t|^k)e^{t\Re(\lambda)}\|x\|,$$

where $k = \alpha(\lambda) - 1$, and where $\Re(\lambda)$ denotes the real part of the eigenvalue $\lambda \in \mathbb{C}$. In particular, if A_λ denotes A restricted to E_λ, then

$$\lim_{|t| \to \infty} \frac{\ln(\|e^{tA_\lambda}\|)}{t} = \Re(\lambda).$$

PROOF:

(*i*) follows from the invariance of G_λ under A, hence under e^{tA}.

(*ii*) A fundamental theorem of linear algebra asserts that $\mathbb{C}^n$ is the direct sum of the spaces G_λ:

$$\mathbb{C}^n = \bigoplus_{\lambda \in \Lambda(A)} G_\lambda.$$

Every vector $z \in \mathbb{C}^n$ can then be (uniquely) written as

$$z = \sum_\lambda \psi_\lambda(z),$$

with $\psi_\lambda(z) \in G_\lambda$. Thus, if $x \in \mathbb{R}^n$, $x = \overline{x} = \sum_\lambda \overline{\psi_\lambda(x)}$, and since $\overline{G_\lambda} = G_{\overline{\lambda}}$ (because A has real entries $M_n(\mathbb{R})$) it follows that

$$\psi_{\overline{\lambda}}(x) = \overline{\psi_\lambda(x)}.$$

This proves that $\Re(\psi_\lambda(x)) \in E_\lambda$ and, since $x = \sum_\lambda \Re(\psi_\lambda(x))$, $\mathbb{R}^n$ is the direct sum of the spaces E_λ.

(*iii*) All the norms being equivalents, it suffices to show (*iii*) for a particular norm. Let $|\cdot|$ be the usual norm on $\mathbb{C}^n$ defined as $|z|^2 = \sum_{i=1}^n z_i \overline{z_i}$ and $\|\cdot\|$ the norm on $\mathbb{C}^n$ defined by $\|z\| = \sum_\lambda |\psi_\lambda(z)|$.

For $z \in G_\lambda$,

$$e^{tA} z = e^{\lambda t} e^{tA - t\lambda I} z,$$

and

$$e^{tA - t\lambda I} z = \sum_{k=0}^{\alpha(\lambda)-1} t^k \frac{(A - \lambda I)^k}{k!} z,$$

because $(A - \lambda I)^k z = 0$ for $k \geq \alpha(\lambda)$. Thus $e^{tA} z = e^{t\lambda} P(t) z$ where $P(t) \in M_n(\mathbb{C})$ is a polynomial in t whose degree is $< \alpha(\lambda)$. Therefore, there exists a constant C such that for all $t \in \mathbb{R}$ and $z \in G_\lambda$

$$\|e^{tA} z\| \leq C(1 + |t|^{\alpha(\lambda)-1}) e^{t\Re(\lambda)} \|z\|.$$

Replacing z by $e^{-tA} z$ in this formula, and t by $-t$, one also deduces that

$$\|e^{tA} z\| \geq \frac{1}{C(1 + |t|^{\alpha(\lambda)-1})} e^{t\Re(\lambda)} \|z\|.$$

If now $x \in E_\lambda$, set $z = \psi_\lambda(x)$. If λ is real $z = x$. If λ has an imaginary part $x = z + \overline{z}$. In this latter case $\|x\| = 2\|z\|$ and

$$\|e^{tA} x\| = \|e^{tA} z\| + \|\overline{e^{tA} z}\| = 2\|e^{tA} z\|.$$

One then obtains the desired result by replacing z by x and C by $2C$ in the previous inequalities. $\square$

11.1.1   Hyperbolic matrices, sources, sinks and saddles

The matrix A is called **hyperbolic** if its eigenvalues have nonzero real parts. Suppose that A is hyperbolic and set $\Lambda^+(A) = \{\lambda \in \Lambda(A) : \Re(\lambda) > 0\}$ and $\Lambda^-(A) = \{\lambda \in \Lambda(A) : \Re(\lambda) < 0\}$. Then

$$\Lambda(A) = \Lambda^+(A) \cup \Lambda^-(A),$$

and according to proposition 11.1.3,

$$\mathbb{R}^n = E^u \bigoplus E^s,$$

with

$$E^u = \bigoplus_{\lambda \in \Lambda^+(A)} E_\lambda,$$

and

$$E^s = \bigoplus_{\lambda \in \Lambda^-(A)} E_\lambda.$$

Such a decomposition is invariant under e^{tA}. Furthermore, assuming that, $0 < a < \min_{\Lambda^-(A)} |\Re(\lambda)|$ and $0 < b < \min_{\Lambda^+(A)} \Re(\lambda)$, there exists $C > 0$ such that for all $t > 0$

$$\forall x \in E^s : \|e^{tA}x\| \leq Ce^{-at}\|x\| \tag{11.2}$$

and

$$\forall x \in E^u : \|e^{-tA}x\| \leq Ce^{-bt}\|x\|. \tag{11.3}$$

Sources, sinks and saddles

The origin $0 \in \mathbb{R}^n$ is called
- a *source* if $\mathbb{R}^n = E^u$,
- a *sink* if $\mathbb{R}^n = E^s$,
- a *saddle* if $\mathbb{R}^n = E^u \bigoplus E^s$ with $E^s \neq \{0\}$ and $E^u \neq \{0\}$.

If 0 is a saddle, the sets E^s and E^u are called, respectively, the stable space and the unstable space.

Remark 11.1.4 If 0 is a sink, inequality 11.2 shows that for t large enough Φ_t is a contraction and 0 is a global attractor, in the sense of the definition given in section 10.6.

The following proposition shows that it is always possible to choose a norm on $\mathbb{R}^n$ such that Φ_t is a contraction for **all** $t > 0$. Such a norm is called an *adapted norm*. A proof can be found in [149].

Proposition 11.1.5 *Let* $0 < a < \min_{\Lambda^-(A)} |\Re(\lambda)|$ *and* $0 < b < \min_{\Lambda^+(A)} \Re(\lambda)$. *The exists a norm* $\|.\|$ *on* $\mathbb{R}^n$ *such that for all* $t > 0$

$$\forall x \in E^s : \|e^{tA}x\| \leq e^{-at}\|x\|,$$

and

$$\forall x \in E^u : \ \|e^{-tA}x\| \leq e^{-bt}\|x\|.$$

11.1.2 Two dimensional linear systems

We suppose here that $n = 2$. Let

$$A = \begin{pmatrix} a & b \\ c & d \end{pmatrix},$$

and let λ_1, λ_2 be the eigenvalues (possibly equals) of A. The related trace and determinant are given by

$$T = \lambda_1 + \lambda_2 = a + d,$$

and

$$D = \lambda_1 \lambda_2 = ad - bc.$$

Furthermore, let

$$\Delta = T^2 - 4D$$

be the discriminant of the characteristic polynomial of A. The nature of the origin easily follows from the signs of T and D:

- If $D < 0$, the eigenvalues are real of opposite signs, and the origin is a saddle.

- If $D > 0$ and $T < 0$ (respectively $T > 0$), the eigenvalues have negative real parts and 0 is a sink (respectively a source). In this latter case, there are two distinct situations:

(i) If $\Delta > 0$, the eigenvalues are real.

(ii) If $\Delta < 0$, the eigenvalues are complex conjugates and 0 is called a spiral sink or a spiral source.

- If $D > 0$ and $T = 0$, the eigenvalues are $i\omega$ and $-i\omega$ for some $\omega \in \mathbb{R}$. The trajectories are then periodic with period $2\pi/\omega$ and the origin is called a *center*.

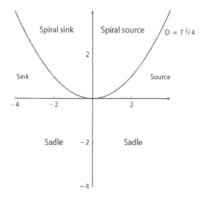

FIGURE 11.1: Nature of the origin in the plane (trace, determinant).

Example 11.1.6 A saddle

$$A = \begin{pmatrix} 1 & 1 \\ 0 & -1 \end{pmatrix}.$$

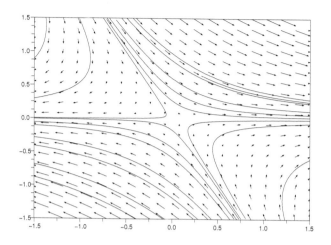

FIGURE 11.2: A saddle.

Example 11.1.7 A sink

$$A = \begin{pmatrix} -2 & 0 \\ 1 & -3 \end{pmatrix}.$$

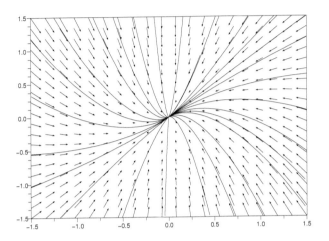

FIGURE 11.3: A sink.

Example 11.1.8 A spiral sink

$$A = \begin{pmatrix} -1 & -1 \\ 2 & 0 \end{pmatrix}.$$

11.2   Linearization and stable manifolds

Let F be a C^k vector field with $k \geq 1$. If p is an equilibrium, F can be rewritten in a neighbourhood of p as

$$F(x) = A(x - p) + o(x - p),$$

where $A = DF(p)$. Thus, letting $y = x - p$, the differential equation (9.4) takes the form

$$\dot{y} = Ay + o(y).$$

It is then natural to compare the trajectories of (9.4) in the neighbourhood of p with the trajectories of the linearized system. We will see here that, when

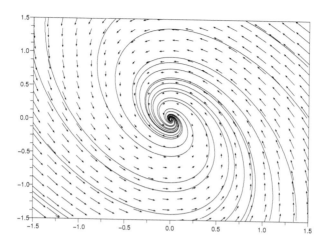

FIGURE 11.4: A spiral sink.

A is hyperbolic, the local behaviour of (9.4) near p is given by the linearized system

$$\dot{y} = Ay.$$

Equilibrium p is called hyperbolic if $A = \mathrm{D}F(p)$ is an hyperbolic matrix. It is called a source (respectively a sink or a saddle) if the origin is a source (respectively a sink or a saddle) of the linearized equation.

11.2.1 Nonlinear sinks

Proposition 11.2.1 *Suppose that p is a sink for a C^1 vector field F. Let $A = \mathrm{D}F(p)$. Then for all $0 < a < \min_{\lambda \in A} |\Re(\lambda)|$ there exists a norm $\|.\|$ and a neighbourhood U of p such that for all $x \in U$ and $t \geq 0$*

$$\|\Phi_t(x) - p\| \leq e^{-at}\|x - p\|.$$

In particular, p is an attractor.

Proof:

Suppose $p = 0$. Write $F(x) = Ax + \|x\|\varepsilon(x)$ with $\varepsilon(0) = 0$ and ε continuous. Let $t \mapsto x(t)$ be the solution to (9.4) and $h(t) = \|x(t)\|\varepsilon(x(t))$. Therefore, for all $t \geq 0$,

$$x(t) = e^{tA}\left(\int_0^t e^{-sA}h(s)\mathrm{d}s + x(0)\right).$$

Fix $a < b < \min |\Re(\lambda)|$. Then, by proposition (11.1.5)

$$\|x(t)\| \le \left(\int_0^t e^{-(t-s)b} \|h(s)\| ds + e^{-bt} \|x(0)\|, \right.$$

for a certain norm $\|.\|$. Set $v(t) = e^{bt} \|x(t)\|$. Thus

$$v(t) \le \int_0^t v(s) \|\varepsilon(x(s))\| ds + \|x(0)\|.$$

Let now $r > 0$ be such that $\|x\| \le r \Rightarrow \|\varepsilon(x)\| \le b - a$. Then, by Gronwall's lemma

$$v(t) \le e^{(b-a)t} \|x(0)\| \le e^{(b-a)t} r,$$

as long as $\|x(t)\| \le r$. It then follows that

$$\|x(t)\| \le e^{-at} \|x(0)\| \le r,$$

for all $t \ge 0$ and $x \in B(0, r)$.

$\square$

11.2.2 The stable manifold theorem

Let p be an equilibrium and U a neighbourhood of p. The *(global) stable manifold* of p is the set

$$W^s(p) = \{x \in \mathbb{R}^n; \omega(x) = p\},$$

and the *(local) stable manifold* of p is the set

$$W^s_U(p) = \{x \in U \ : \ \forall t \ge 0, \Phi_t(x) \in U\} \cap W^s(p).$$

Note that $W^s_U(p)$ is not (in general) the intersection of U and $W^s(p)$ because there may exist points arbitrarily close to p which converge to p after leaving U (see figure 11.6). The global (respectively local) unstable manifold is defined analogously as the global (resp. local) stable manifold of the reversed flow $\Psi_t = \Psi_{-t}$.

The following theorem is known as the *Stable Manifold Theorem*. The interested reader will find detailed proofs in classical reference books such as [79] or [149].

Theorem 11.2.2 *Let F be a C^k, $k \ge 1$ vector field and p an hyperbolic equilibrium. There exists a neighbourhood U of p and a C^k map $H : E^s \cap U \to E^u$ such that*

(i) $W^s_U(p) = \{x \in U \ : \ \forall t \ge 0, \Phi_t(x) \in U\}$,

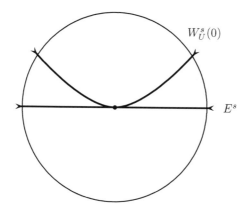

FIGURE 11.5: A local stable manifold.

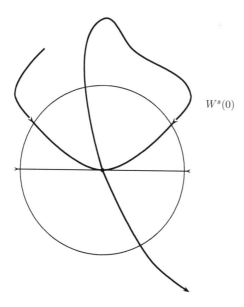

FIGURE 11.6: The global stable manifold is not a submanifold.

(ii) $H(0) = 0, DH(0) = 0$ *and*

$$W_U^s(p) = \{p + (u, H(u)) :: u \in E^s \cap U\}.$$

Let us briefly comment on this result. If p is a sink, $W_U^s = U$. If p is a saddle, W_U^s is the graph of a C^k map tangent to p at the stable space. It is the *submanifold* of U having dimension $\dim(E^s)$ whose tangent space at p is E^s. Note also that every trajectory based at $x \in U \setminus W_U^s(p)$ leaves U at some time $t > 0$. The global stable manifold can be rewritten as

$$W^s(p) = \cup_{t>0} \Phi_{-t}(W_U^s(p)).$$

This makes $W^s(p)$ an abstract *submanifold* (or an *immersion*) but not necessarily a submanifold of $\mathbb{R}^n$.

Example 11.2.3 Let

$$\begin{cases} \dot{x} = 2y, \\ \dot{y} = 2x - 3x^2. \end{cases}$$

At $(0,0)$

$$DF(0,0) = \begin{pmatrix} 0 & 2 \\ 2 & 0 \end{pmatrix}$$

of eigenvalues 2 and -2. The associated eigenvectors are $(1,1)$ and $(-1,1)$. The origin is therefore an hyperbolic equilibrium. The map

$$H(x, y) = y^2 + x^3 - x^2,$$

is constant along trajectories. It then easily follows that

(i) $W^s(0,0) = W^u(0,0) = \{(x,y) \in \mathbb{R}^2 : y^2 + x^3 - x^2 = 0\}$.

(ii) For U small enough

$$W_U^u(0,0) = \{(x,y) \in U : y = x\sqrt{1-x}\},$$

and

$$W_U^s(0,0) = \{(x,y) \in U : y = -x\sqrt{1-x}\}.$$

Stable and unstable local manifolds are clearly C^1 submanifolds (being graphs of C^1 functions) while the global stable manifold has a singularity at $(0,0)$ (a double point), and is not a submanifold of $\mathbb{R}^2$.

11.2.3 The Hartmann-Grobman linearization theorem[*]

Another useful theorem allowing us to understand the local behaviour of the dynamics in the neighbourhood of an hyperbolic equilibrium is the *Linearisation Theorem* of Hartmann and Grobman. In words this theorem just says that the dynamics in the neighbourhood of an hyperbolic equilibrium looks like (up to a continuous change of variable) the dynamics of the linearised system. In more mathematical terms, it says:

Theorem 11.2.4 *Let F be a C^1 vector field and p an hyperbolic equilibrium. There exist neighbourhoods U of $0 \in \mathbb{R}^n$, V of p, and an homeomorphism (i.e. a bi-continuous invertible function) $H : U \to V$ such that*

$$\Phi_t(H(x)) = H(e^{tA}x),$$

for all t such that $e^{tA}x \in U$.

11.2.4 The May and Leonard model (the end)

We can now rigorously prove proposition 10.2.5 on the May and Leonard system (see section 10.2.2). We proceed in three steps.

Step (i). Existence of an heteroclinic cycle $\Gamma : e_1 \hookrightarrow e_2 \hookrightarrow e_3 \hookrightarrow e_1$. Consider the two species systems (1 and 2) given by equation (10.2). From the previous analysis we know that for all $x > 0$ and $y > 0$ the solution to (10.2) based at (x, y) converges toward e_2. Furthermore, e_1 is an hyperbolic saddle whose stable manifold is the x-axis. The local unstable manifold at e_1, $W^s_{loc}(e_1)$ is thus a curve which meets the half plane $x > 0$. Let $p \in W^s_{loc}(e_1) \cap (\mathbb{R}^*_+)^2$. Then $\alpha(p) = e_1$ and $\omega(p) = e_2$. This implies that $e_1 \hookrightarrow e_2$ and, from symmetry, $e_1 \hookrightarrow e_2 \hookrightarrow e_3 \hookrightarrow e_1$.

Step (ii). For all $p \in E \setminus \Delta$, $\omega(p) \subset \Gamma$. We follow here Hofbauer and Sigmund [87]. First remark that the origin is an hyperbolic source for (10.1). By proposition 11.2.1 there exists a neighbourhood U of the origin such that $E \setminus U$ is positively invariant. Let $S, P : E \to \mathbb{R}$ and $Q : E \setminus U \to \mathbb{R}$ be the functions defined by

$$S = x + y + z, \ P = xyz \text{ and } Q = \frac{P}{S^3}.$$

An easy computation shows that

(i) $\dot{S} \leq S(1 - S)$;

(ii) $\dot{P} = P(3 - (1 + \alpha + \beta)S)$;

(iii)

$$\dot{Q} = S^{-4} P (1 - \frac{\alpha + \beta}{2}) [(x - y)^2 + (y - z)^2 + (z - x)^2].$$

From (i) one deduces that the set $\{(x, y, z) \in E : S \leq 1\}$ attracts all the trajectories and that the system is dissipative. From (iii) one deduces, by application of corollary 10.5.2, that for $\alpha + \beta < 2$ and $p \in E \backslash \Delta$, $\omega(p) \in \partial E \cup \Delta$. Since $Q = 1/9$ on *Delta* and $\dot{Q} < 0$ outside $\partial E \cup \Delta$, $\omega(p) \in \partial E$. Since 0 is an hyperbolic source, $\omega(p) \subset \partial E \backslash \{0\}$. Let $q = (q_1, q_2, q_3) \in \omega(p)$. Because $q \in \partial E$ one can suppose $q_3 = 0$. Hence $q \in \{e_1, e_2\}$, $\omega(q) = e_2$ and $\alpha(q) = e_1$. This proves that $q \in \Gamma$.

Remark 11.2.5 The proof above also show that for $\alpha + \beta > 2$ the system is persistent.

Step (iii). For all $p \in \text{int}(E) \backslash \Delta$, $\omega(p) = \Gamma$.

We know that $\omega(p)$ contains one of the equilibria e_1, e_2 or e_3. Suppose $e_1 \in \omega(p)$ and let V be a neighbourhood of e_1 as in the Hartman-Grobman theorem. The trajectory based at p meets V infinitely often, and by the Hartman-Grobman theorem, it leaves V in the neighbourhood of the unstable manifold of e_1. This shows that this unstable manifold meets $\omega(p)$. By invariance it follows that $e_2 \in \omega(p)$ and, by symmetry, $e_3 \in \omega(p)$. Since $\omega(p)$ is connected, $\omega(p) = \Gamma$.

Part IV

Linear noise approximation

Chapter 12

Density dependent population processes and the linear noise approximation

We present an important family of Markov chains appearing naturally in many modelling frameworks, like epidemic theory or chemical reaction network dynamics. It is often impossible to get analytical results on the solutions of master equations associated with large and complicated gene network dynamics, and scientists rely most of the time on simulations. This is a good solution for getting ideas of what is going on in specific networks, but it is less useful to gather conceptual results. The linear noise approximation method provides a way of obtaining useful information through gaussian approximation: one can then consider the covariance matrix and try to understand noise sources, or to optimize network parameters to obtain required noise levels.

12.1 A law of large numbers

We follow the presentation of [47], trying to explain the limiting properties of such dynamics in a simple way. When adapted to chemical reaction networks, the resulting asymptotic approximation is known as **the linear noise approximation**; see [43] (as developed in [178] [179]), and [180], among others. We focus on families of Markov chains of a particular kind, which depend on parameter N which can be interpreted in different contexts, like total population size or volume. Within our modelling framework, N can be seen as a typical steady state value of some gene product, which is assumed to be large. We begin with an example: consider a simple chemical reaction of the form

$$A + B \longrightarrow C,$$

where the interaction of one molecule of type A with one molecule of type B produces one molecule of type C. Let $X(t) = (X_A(t), X_B(t), X_C(t))$ be the random process describing the time evolution of the number of A, B and C molecules. At time $t = 0$, the abundances are given by $X_A(0)$, $X_B(0)$ and $X_C(0)$, with $N = X_A(0) + X_B(0) + X_C(0)$. We assume that the reaction is governed by the **law of mass action**, which states that the probability that a molecule of type A meets and interacts with a type B molecule is proportional to the concentration of B molecules. Hence, the probability that a C molecule is created in the small time interval $(t, t + h)$, $h \approx 0$, is on the order of $h\mu X_A(t) X_B(t)/N$. The related Markov chain is not irreducible since both $X_A(t)$ and $X_B(t)$ are nonincreasing functions of t. This is our starting example of a density dependent population process. We will come to more biologically interesting models in what follows. The time evolution of $X(t)$ is particular, since, assuming that there is a single transition in the time interval $(t, t + h)$,

$$X(t + h) = X(t) + (-1, -1, 1),$$

which occurs at rate $h\beta(X(t)) = h\mu X_A(t) X_B(t)/N$ (see (2.4)). More generally,

$$X(t) = X(0) + R(t)(-1, -1, 1), \tag{12.1}$$

where $R(t)$ denotes the number of times the reaction has occurred by time t. It turns out that one can express $R(t)$ in a nice probabilistic way using nonhomogeneous Poisson processes; see, e.g., [6] and [47].

In the general situation, a **density dependent population process** models the stochastic evolution of the abundances of a set of species $\mathcal{S} = \{S_1, \cdots, S_M\}$ (see section 3.1), and is defined using nonnegative functions β_l, where $l = (l_1, \cdots, l_M) \in \mathbb{Z}^M$ is an integer valued vector. There is also a variable N which can be chosen in various ways, according to the setting: it might model population size or cell volume. $X(t)$ is a random vector

$$X(t) = (X_1(t), \cdots, X_M(t)) \in \mathbb{N}^M,$$

where the $X_i(t)$ counts the number of individuals of type i present in the population at time t. Assuming that $X(t) = x$, one considers only transitions of the form

$$x \longrightarrow x + l, \ l \in \mathbb{Z}^M,$$

of rate

$$q_{x,x+l} = W_l(x) = N\beta_l\left(\frac{x}{N}\right), \tag{12.2}$$

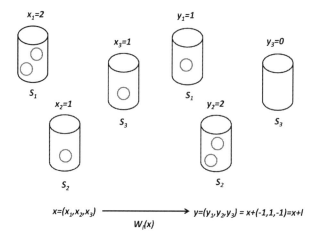

FIGURE 12.1: During a small time interval $(t, t + h)$, the system jumps from $X(t) = x$ to $X(t + h) = y = x + l$, where $l = (-1, 1, -1)$, meaning that this reaction consumes one molecule of type S_1 and one molecule of type S_3 to produce one molecule of type S_2.

where W_l is the propensity function which was defined in section 3.1. The stoichiometric matrix has columns given by the vectors $l \in \mathbb{Z}^M$ for which the propensity function $W_l(x) = q_{x,x+l}$ is positive. Figure 12.1 provides a simple example of such transitions.

Here, the transition rates depend on the actual state $X(t) = x$ only through the **ratio or concentration** x/N. Let

$$\bar{X}_N(t) = \frac{X(t)}{N} \in \mathbb{R}_+^M.$$

In the above example, $l = (-1, -1, 1)$ and $\beta_l(\bar{X}_N) = \mu(X_A/N)(X_B/N) = \mu \bar{X}_A \bar{X}_B$. One likewise defines the related transition rates as

$$q_{\bar{x}, \bar{y}}^N = N \beta_{N(\bar{y} - \bar{x})}(\bar{x}),$$

where $l = N(\bar{y} - \bar{x}) \in \mathbb{Z}$, when both $\bar{x}$ and $\bar{y}$ are concentrations of the form k/N for $k \in \mathbb{N}^M$. The asymptotic behaviour is studied under some mathematical hypotheses. The state space is restricted by fixing a domain E of $\mathbb{R}^M$, and by setting

$$E_N = E \cap \{\frac{x}{N}; \; x \in \mathbb{N}^M\}.$$

The process is forced to stay in E_N by imposing that the transition rate functions β_l are such that $\beta_l(\bar{x}) > 0$, $\bar{x} \in E_N$, implying that $\bar{x} + l/N \in E_N$. The large N limiting process is governed by the following **vector field**:

$$F(\bar{x}) = \sum_l l\beta_l(\bar{x}). \tag{12.3}$$

Notice that for small $h > 0$,

$$Nh\beta_l(\bar{x}) \approx P(\bar{X}_N(t+h) - \bar{X}_N(t) = \frac{l}{N}|\bar{X}_N(t) = \bar{x}),$$

so that

$$\begin{aligned} hF(\bar{x}) &\approx \sum_l \frac{l}{N}P(\bar{X}_N(t+h) - \bar{X}_N(t) = \frac{l}{N}|\bar{X}_N(t) = \bar{x}) \\ &= \mathbb{E}(\bar{X}_N(t+h) - \bar{X}_N(t)|\bar{X}_N(t) = \bar{x}) \end{aligned}$$

is approximatively the conditional mean increment of the process $\bar{X}_N(t)$ given that $\bar{X}_N(t) = \bar{x}$.

Law of large numbers for density dependent population processes

Theorem 12.1.1 *[47] Suppose that for each compact set $K \subset E$*

$$\sum_l |l| \sup_{\bar{x} \in K} \beta_l(\bar{x}) < \infty,$$

and that there exists a constant M^K such that

$$|F(\bar{y}) - F(\bar{x})| \leq M^K|\bar{y} - \bar{x}|, \quad \bar{x}, \bar{y} \in K.$$

Assume furthermore that $\bar{X}_N(0) \longrightarrow x_0$ as $N \to \infty$. Let $\bar{X}(t)$ be the solution to the following equation:

$$\bar{X}(t) = x_0 + \int_0^t F(\bar{X}(s))\mathrm{d}s. \tag{12.4}$$

Then, for any $t \geq 0$,

$$\lim_{N\to\infty} \sup_{s\leq t} |\bar{X}_N(s) - \bar{X}(s)| = 0. \tag{12.5}$$

Theorem 12.1.1 provides a way of approximating the behaviour of the concentration process $\bar{X}_N(t)$ when N is large: it states basically that $\bar{X}_N(s)$,

$s \leq t$, is well described by the solution to the (deterministic or nonrandom) ordinary differential equation

$$\frac{\mathrm{d}\bar{X}(s)}{\mathrm{d}s} = F(\bar{X}(s)), s \leq t, \tag{12.6}$$

$\bar{X}(0) = x_0$. The above approximation then yields the intuitive relation

$$\bar{X}(s+h) - \bar{X}(s) \approx hF(\bar{X}(s)) \approx \mathbb{E}(\bar{X}_N(t+h) - \bar{X}_N(t)|\bar{X}_N(t) = \bar{X}(s)),$$

when $h \approx 0$ and $N \gg 1$.

For our basic example, one obtains the limiting o.d.e.

$$\frac{\mathrm{d}\bar{X}_A}{\mathrm{d}t} = -\mu\bar{X}_A\bar{X}_B, \quad \frac{\mathrm{d}\bar{X}_B}{\mathrm{d}t} = -\mu\bar{X}_A\bar{X}_B \text{ and } \frac{\mathrm{d}\bar{X}_C}{\mathrm{d}t} = \mu\bar{X}_A\bar{X}_B.$$

Sketch of proof of theorem 12.1.1*

We restrict the heuristic explanation to the above example; the general case is given in [47]. The stochastic process $R(t)$ given in (12.1) is

$$R(t) = Y(N\int_0^t \beta(\frac{X(s)}{N})\mathrm{d}s),$$

where Y is a unit Poisson process. This kind of representation of time-continuous Markov chains is used, among other things, to prove limiting theorems or to unify various kind of simulations algorithms; see, e.g., [6]. Looking at concentrations, one gets

$$\begin{aligned}\bar{X}_N(t) &= \bar{X}_N(0) + \frac{1}{N}Y(N\int_0^t \beta(\bar{X}_N(s))\mathrm{d}s)\ (-1,-1,1)\\ &= \bar{X}_N(0) + \int_0^t \beta(\bar{X}_N(s))\mathrm{d}s\ (-1,-1,1)\\ &\quad + \frac{1}{N}\left(Y(N\int_0^t \beta(\bar{X}_N(s))\mathrm{d}s) - N\int_0^t \beta(\bar{X}_N(s))\mathrm{d}s\right)(-1,-1,1)\end{aligned}$$

where we have substracted the mean of the Poisson process in the second term. Poisson process theory provides the following law of large numbers:

$$\lim_{N\to\infty} \sup_{u \leq u_0} |\frac{Y(Nu)}{N} - u| = 0,$$

$\forall u_0 > 0$. This motivates the result of theorem 12.1.1 since the above estimates show that

$$\bar{X}_N(t) \approx \bar{X}_N(0) + \int_0^t \beta(\bar{X}_N(s))\mathrm{d}s\ (-1,-1,1).$$

12.2   Illustration: bistable behaviour of self-regulated genes

Chapter 1 introduces a self-regulated gene where dimers bind to the promoter (see figure 1.1), realizing in this way a feedback loop. Positive feedback loops can lead to bistability, as illustrated in figure 1.6. Mathematically, one can provide an exact analytical formula for the related steady state distribution using the method of transfer matrices; see section A.3 or [58] and [57]. In principle, one should be able to use these mathematical formulas to check bistability: we, however, follow [104], using several approximations which lead to a simple mathematical expression. We will see that a positive feedback coupled to dimerization can induce bistability. We hence assume that protein monomers first form protein dimers before binding to the promoter.

Let N be a large parameter which describes a large steady state expression. Adopting the law of mass action, one can suppose that

$$g(n) \sim n\frac{n}{N} = (\frac{n}{N})^2 N.$$

The product $n(n/N)$ models mass action kinetics, where a particular molecule interacts with any molecule with a rate equal or proportional to the related concentration. Likewise, we assume that

$$\kappa = \bar{\kappa}N, \quad \mu_1 = N\bar{\mu}_1, \quad \mu_0 = N\bar{\mu}_0,$$

for some positive constants $\bar{\kappa}$, $\bar{\mu}_0$ and $\bar{\mu}_1$. When the promoter is fast, the quasi-equilibrium approximation leads to a birth and death process of birth rate

$$\lambda_n = \frac{\kappa(n)\mu_0 + g(n)\mu_1}{\kappa(n) + g(n)} = N\frac{\bar{\kappa}\bar{\mu}_0 + (\frac{n}{N})^2\bar{\mu}_1}{\bar{\kappa} + (\frac{n}{N})^2},$$

and death rate

$$\nu_n = \nu n = N\nu\frac{n}{N};$$

see example 2.4.1. The large volume approximation shows that the behaviour of the system is well described by the o.d.e. based on

$$F(\bar{x}) = \sum_{l=-1,+1} l\beta_l(\bar{x}) = \frac{\bar{\kappa}\bar{\mu}_0 + \bar{x}^2\bar{\mu}_1}{\bar{\kappa} + \bar{x}^2} - \nu\bar{x}.$$

The authors of [104] observed that F is a gradient vector field (see exercise 10.5.4)

$$F(\bar{x}) = -\nabla\Phi(x),$$

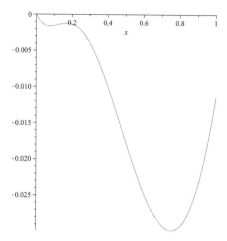

FIGURE 12.2: The potential function (12.7) describing the o.d.e. associated with the expression of a self-regulated gene. The potential has two equilibria, which might correspond in some way to the two modes of the bimodal steady state distribution.

for the Lyapunov function

$$\Phi(x) = \frac{\nu x^2}{2} - \bar{\mu}_1 x + (\bar{\mu}_1 - \bar{\mu}_0)\sqrt{\kappa}\arctan(\frac{x}{\sqrt{\kappa}}). \tag{12.7}$$

Corollary 10.5.2 and example 10.5.4 show that the orbits converge toward the minima of Φ. Figure 12.2 shows a numerical example where the system is bistable, with two equilibria, which might correspond to the two modes of the related steady state distribution.

12.3 Epigenetics and multistationarity

The central dogma of molecular biology, *gene → mRNA → protein*, results in traits which are associated to **phenotypes**. Waddington [182] proposed that genes are not the sole actors of trait inheritance, and defined an **epigenetic landscape model** where traits are stored in attractors of dynamical systems associated with gene regulatory networks. This picture permits to shed light on the nonobvious existing relations between genes and traits; see, e.g., [91].

The self-regulated gene model of chapter 1 can already store two modes in its stationary distribution; see, e.g., figures 1.5 and 1.6, or the o.d.e. of section 12.2, which has been obtained from the linear noise approximation. Such modes define two significantly different expression levels, which might correspond to different phenotypes; see, e.g., [92], [134] or [46]. A typical example was presented in section 5.13, where the bistable switch associated with the lytic and lysogenic modes leads to two different phenotypes; see, e.g., the discussion in [7]. More generally, if a Markov chain $X(t) = (X_1(t), \cdots, X_M(t))$ describes the time evolution of the abundances of species S_i, $i = 1, \cdots, M$, the possible traits should be stored in the modes of the associated steady state distribution, or in the multiple equilibria of the related o.d.e., as provided in section 12.1. The linear noise approximation assumes propensity functions of the form $W_l(x) = N\beta_l(x/N)$ for a large parameter N, and arrives at the o.d.e. (12.6)

$$\frac{d\bar{X}(t)}{dt} = F(\bar{X}(t)), t \geq 0,$$

where the vector field F is

$$F(\bar{x}) = \sum_l l\beta_l(\bar{x}).$$

The natural question is then to find conditions of F ensuring multiple equilibria. The author of [170] conjectured that a necessary condition for the existence of multiple equilibria is the existence of a positive feedback loop: this is the well-known **Thomas conjecture**; see also [100] and [171]. This question has been approached in [161] using the so-called **interaction graph** associated with the Jacobian matrix of F, using the results of [64] on univalence of mappings; see also [176], [123] and [99], or the more recent paper of [129], the latter giving some historical data.

We follow [161]. An interaction graph $\mathcal{G} = (V, \mathcal{E}, \text{sgn})$ of nodes set V and of directed edge set $\mathcal{E}$ is a finite directed graph $(V, \mathcal{E})$ where a sign map, sgn : $\mathcal{E} \longrightarrow \{-1, +1\}$ assigns -1 or $+1$ to every directed edge $e = (e_- \to e_+)$ of $\mathcal{E}$. A circuit c is a sequence of edges $e^1, \cdots, e^k$ such that $e_-^{i+1} = e_+^i$, $i = 1, \cdots, k-1$, and $e_+^l = e_-^1$. The sign of a circuit c is

$$\text{sgn}(c) = \prod_{e \in c} \text{sgn}(e).$$

A circuit c is **positive** when $\text{sgn}(c) = +1$. Let A be square matrix of size M. The interaction graph associated with A, denoted by $\mathcal{G}(A)$, is the interaction graph of node set $V = \{1, \cdots, M\}$, and of edge set $\mathcal{E}$, where $e = (i \to j) \in \mathcal{E}$ if and only if $a_{ij} \neq 0$. The associated sign function is such that $\text{sgn}(e) = \text{sgn}(a_{ij})$.

Coming back to the Thomas conjecture, let F be a differentiable map $F : \mathbb{R}^M \longrightarrow \mathbb{R}^M$ of Jacobian matrix DF. The related interaction graph mapping associates to each $a \in \mathbb{R}^M$ the interaction graph $\mathcal{G}(DF(a))$, where the sign function is

$$\text{sgn}(e) = \text{sgn}(\frac{\partial F_i(a)}{\partial x_j}), \quad \text{for } e = (i \to j),$$

when the above partial derivative does not vanish at a. Assume that F is defined on I, which is a product of open intervals I_i, $i = 1, \cdots, M$, where each interval I_i is of the form $I_i =]a_i, b_i[$. The following theorem has been proven in [161]:

Theorem 12.3.1 (Thomas conjecture) *Assume that I is open and that F has at least two nondegenerate zeroes in I. Then, there exists $a \in I$ such that the associated interaction graph $\mathcal{G}(DF(a))$ contains a positive circuit.*

This provides the basis for understanding the role of positive feedback loops in gene networks; see, e.g., the discussion in section 5.12. The author of [161] proved this theorem by rewriting the determinant of the Jacobian matrix as a product of cyclic permutations, which are mapped toward circuits. Similar works have been performed for chemical reaction networks or mass action kinetics, where F takes specific mathematical forms, by, among others, [31], [93] and [94], where these works use different kinds of graphical methods; see also [129]. More recent results on instabilities and univalence of chemical reaction networks can be found in, among others, [33], [34], [128], [35], [186], [42], [32] or [88].

12.4   Gaussian approximation

The fluctuation

$$V_N(t) = \sqrt{N}(\bar{X}_N(t) - \bar{X}(t)), \tag{12.8}$$

is asymptotically distributed according to a Gaussian law; see, e.g., [47], that is

$$\bar{X}_N(t) \approx \bar{X}(t) + \frac{V(t)}{\sqrt{N}},$$

where the limiting gaussian process $V(t)$ is defined using the **Jacobian** $\mathrm{D}F(\bar{x}) = (\partial F_i(\bar{x})/\partial \bar{x}_j)$: one first considers the time-nonhomogeneous matrix valued differential equation

$$\frac{\partial \phi(t, s)}{\partial t} = \mathrm{D}F(\bar{X}(t))\phi(t, s), \tag{12.9}$$

where $\phi(s, s) = \mathrm{id}$, and id is the identity matrix. Notice that (12.9) is the linearisation of the o.d.e. (12.4). Let

$$G(\bar{x}) = \sum_l ll^T \beta_l(\bar{x}), \tag{12.10}$$

where A^T denotes the matrix transpose of any matrix A. A nonelementary computation shows that the limiting process has a covariance and a mean given by

$$\mathrm{Cov}(V(t), V(r)) = \int_0^{\min\{t, r\}} \phi(t, s)G(\bar{X}(s))\phi(r, s)^T \mathrm{d}s, \tag{12.11}$$

and

$$\mathbb{E}(V(t)) = \phi(t, 0)V(0); $$

see [47]. The covariance function given in (12.11), $\Sigma(t) = \mathrm{Cov}(V(t), V(t))$, is the solution of the **time-continuous Lyapunov equation**

$$\frac{\mathrm{d}\Sigma(t)}{\mathrm{d}t} = \mathrm{D}F(\bar{X}(t))\Sigma(t) + \Sigma(t)\mathrm{D}F(\bar{X}(t))^T + G(\bar{X}(t)). \tag{12.12}$$

We will use these limiting results in section 12.5.

Multivariate gaussian distribution

A random variable $X \in \mathbb{R}$ is normally distributed if its density is of the form

$$f(x) = \frac{1}{\sqrt{2\pi}\sigma} \exp(-\frac{(x-\mu)^2}{2\sigma^2}),$$

where $\mu \in \mathbb{R}$ is the mean of X and σ^2 is the variance of X. The standard normal distribution is obtained by setting $\mu = 0$ and $\sigma = 1$. A random vector $X = (X_1, \cdots, X_n)^T \in \mathbb{R}^n$ is gaussian or normal multivariate when, for all vectors $b \in \mathbb{R}^n$, the random variable $U = b^T X \in \mathbb{R}$ is normally distributed. If X is multivariate normal, then, for any (p, n) matrix A and any vector $C \in \mathbb{R}^p$, the random vector $Y = AX + C$ is normal multivariate. Let $\mu = \mathbb{E}(X)$ and $\Sigma = \mathrm{Cov}(X)$. Then

$$\mathbb{E}(Y) = A\mathbb{E}(X) + C \text{ and } \mathrm{Cov}(Y) = A\Sigma A^T.$$

X is uniquely characterised by the pair (μ, Σ). When the symmetric covariance matrix Σ is positive definite, the gaussian vector X has the density

$$f(x) = \frac{1}{(2\pi)^{n/2}} \frac{1}{\sqrt{\det(\Sigma)}} \exp(-\frac{1}{2}(X-\mu)^T \Sigma^{-1}(X-\mu)).$$

The related contour lines are ellipsoids since the quadratic form which appears in the density is positive definite. Figure 12.3 provides a plot of the bivariate normal density for $\mu = \mathbb{E}(X) = (1, 1)^T$ and

$$\Sigma = \begin{pmatrix} 2 & 3 \\ 3 & 9 \end{pmatrix}. \tag{12.13}$$

Figure 12.4 shows the plot of a sample of size 100 of this distribution.

Density Plot: Bivariate gaussian distribution

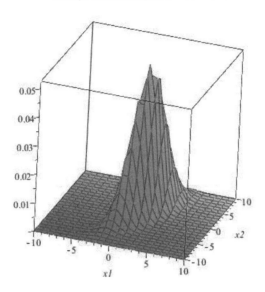

FIGURE 12.3: Plot a normal bivariate density of mean $\mu = (1,1)^T$ and of covariance Σ given by (12.13).

Covariances of random vectors

Let $X = (X_1, \cdots, X_n)^T \in \mathbb{R}^n$ be a random vector, of mean

$$\mathbb{E}(X) = (\mathbb{E}(X_1), \cdots, \mathbb{E}(X_n))^T.$$

The covariance matrix of X is the semi positive definite symmetric (n,n) matrix

$$\begin{aligned} \mathrm{Cov}(X) &= \mathbb{E}((X - \mathbb{E}(X))(X - \mathbb{E}(X))^T \\ &= \mathbb{E}(XX^T) - \mathbb{E}(X)\mathbb{E}(X)^T. \end{aligned}$$

Let $X \in \mathbb{R}^n$ and $Y \in \mathbb{R}^p$ be two random vectors. The cross covariance matrix $\mathrm{Cov}(X,Y)$ associated with X and Y is the (n,p) matrix

$$\mathrm{Cov}(X,Y) = \mathbb{E}((X - \mathbb{E}(X))(Y - \mathbb{E}(Y))^T).$$

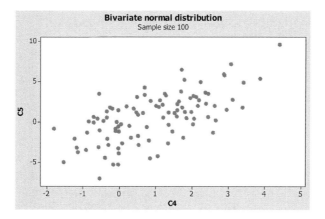

FIGURE 12.4: Sample of size 100 of the bivariate normal distribution described in figure 12.3.

12.4.1 Steady state approximations

Let $\bar{X}_*$ be an asymptotically stable equilibrium of (12.6) such that the eigenvalues of $DF(\bar{X}_*)$ all have negative real parts. In a neighbourhood of $\bar{X}_*$, $\bar{X}(t)$ converges to $\bar{X}_*$; see proposition 11.2.1. The covariance function $\Sigma(t)$ associated with $V(t)$ solves (12.12)

$$\frac{d\Sigma(t)}{dt} = DF(\bar{X}(t))\Sigma(t) + \Sigma(t)DF(\bar{X}(t))^T + G(\bar{X}(t)).$$

Theorem B.2.4 of the Appendix provides sufficient conditions ensuring the convergence of $\Sigma(t)$ to a covariance function Σ solving the **Lyapunov equation**

$$K\Sigma + \Sigma K^T + G(\bar{X}_*) = 0, \qquad (12.14)$$

where we set for convenience

$$K = DF(\bar{X}_*).$$

K is **stable** when all of its eigenvalues have negative real parts. Basically, Σ is the unique positive definite symmetric solution of the above equation when K is stable and G is symmetric and positive definite. The author of [138] arrives at a similar expression using the so-called **fluctuation dissipation theorem**, which is mainly equivalent to the gaussian approximation. Let $\lambda_1, \cdots, \lambda_M$ be the characteristic roots of K, each repeated as often as its multiplicity. One can check that if every sum $\lambda_i + \lambda_k \neq 0$, then Σ is uniquely defined through (12.14) by the symmetric matrix $G(\bar{X}_*)$. The interested reader can consult [105], [63] or section B.2.4 for more mathematical results on this kind of equation.

$G(\bar{X}_*)$ is diagonal when the increments l are such that $l = \pm e_i$, where e_i denotes the ith canonical basis vector of $\mathbb{R}^M$. When, furthermore, $M = 2$, one obtains an exact formula: set

$$\nu_{11} = \frac{-G(\bar{X}_*)_{11}}{2K_{11}} \text{ and } \nu_{22} = \frac{-G(\bar{X}_*)_{22}}{2K_{22}}.$$

Then, according to [173],

$$\Sigma = \Sigma_1 + \Sigma_2, \tag{12.15}$$

where, setting $\triangle = \det(K)$,

$$\Sigma_1 = \nu_{11} \frac{K_{11}}{K_{11} + K_{22}} \left(e_1 e_1^T + \frac{1}{\triangle} \begin{pmatrix} K_{22}^2 & -K_{21}K_{22} \\ -K_{21}K_{22} & K_{21}^2 \end{pmatrix} \right) \tag{12.16}$$

and

$$\Sigma_2 = \nu_{22} \frac{K_{22}}{K_{11} + K_{22}} \left(e_2 e_2^T + \frac{1}{\triangle} \begin{pmatrix} K_{12}^2 & -K_{12}K_{11} \\ -K_{12}K_{11} & K_{11}^2 \end{pmatrix} \right). \tag{12.17}$$

This decomposition will be useful to study noise propagation in simple examples. Figure 12.4 shows the plot of a sample of size 100 of the bivariate normal distribution with $\mu = \mathbb{E}(X) = (1,1)^T$ and of covariance given by (12.13). One sees the emergence of an ellipse, of axes given by the eigenvectors of the covariance matrix.

For arbitrary normal multivariate random vector X, let Y be the projection of X on a line passing through μ, directed by some vector $a \in \mathbb{R}^M$, that is, let

$$Y = \mu + a a^T (X - \mu),$$

and let

$$\mathbb{E}(||X - Y||^2) = \sum_{i=1}^{M} (X_i - Y_i)^2$$

be the mean squared difference. One can show that the latter is minimal when a is a normalised eigenvector associated with the largest eigenvalue of the covariance matrix Σ; see, e.g., [54]. In this case, $\mathbb{E}(X|Y) = Y$, and Y is the best one dimensional approximation of X in the least squared sense. This is the essence of the **linear principal component** method of multivariate analysis, which looks for the best one dimensional approximation of X.

12.5 Illustration: attenuation of noise using negative feedback loops in prokaryotic transcription

We consider the self-regulated gene model of chapter 1, as represented by figures 1.1 and 12.5, with a negative feedback loop, which is realized by the binding of protein dimers on the promoter. Such modules can prevent large fluctuations, and hence are instrumental for gene regulation; see, e.g., [12], [81] or [152]. We take into account mRNAs: the authors of [16] and [124] have shown that, during translation by ribosomes, burst of proteins are released into the cytoplasm, with geometrically distributed sizes. The average burst size b is $b \approx 40$ for LacZ, and $b \approx 5$ for LacA; see, e.g., [103]. The time evolution of this regulatory module was considered through linear first-order networks in [169]; we follow here [173] where, the linear noise approximation is used to understand the effect of negative feedback loops on noise propagation.

Let $X(t) = (X_1(t), X_2(t))^T$ be the state of the system at time t, where $X_1(t)$ is the number of proteins present in the cell at time t and where $X_2(t)$ denotes the number of protein dimers. Then

$$X_1(t) - 2X_2(t) \geq 0$$

gives the number of protein monomers. The authors of [16] and [124] introduce the probability $p(n)$, $n \in \mathbb{N}$, that the protein burst size is n, with

$$p(n) = \frac{b^n}{(1+b)^{n+1}}.$$

Dimerization is modelled by the relation

$$\mathcal{M} + \mathcal{M} \longleftrightarrow \mathcal{D},$$

where the symbols $\mathcal{M}$ and $\mathcal{D}$ represent protein monomers and dimers. Adopting the law of mass action for a cell volume of size N, the rate production of dimers is

$$c_+(X_1 - 2X_2)\frac{(X_1 - 2X_2 - 1)}{N} \tag{12.18}$$

(see section A.1), and the dissociation rate is $c_- X_2$. Furthermore, let α be a decreasing function modelling the negative feedback loop. Transcription and translation are then represented by the set of relations

$$\emptyset \longrightarrow n\mathcal{M}, \ n = 1, \ 2, \cdots \tag{12.19}$$

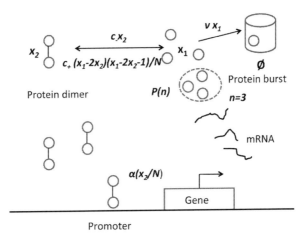

FIGURE 12.5: Bursts of proteins of size n are produced at rate $N\alpha(x_2/N)p(n)$, where x_2 denotes the number of protein dimers, and where α is a decreasing function modelling the negative feedback loop.

which occur at rate $N\alpha(x_2/N)p(n)$. The stoichiometric matrix defined in section 3.1 is given by the infinite matrix

$$A = \begin{pmatrix} -1 & 0 & 0 & 1 & 2 & \cdots & n & n+1 & \cdots \\ 0 & 1 & -1 & 0 & 0 & \cdots & 0 & 0 & \cdots \end{pmatrix}.$$

Recall that the entry a_{ij} associated with species i and reaction j gives the change in copy number of type i molecules when reaction j occurs. In our setting, the first column of A corresponds to the degradation of a monomer, so that the total number of proteins decreases by one. The second column encodes the production of one dimer, and the third one is related to the dissociation of one dimer. The remaining columns encode the various protein burst sizes.

First notice that the transition rate (12.18) is not strictly speaking of the form given in (12.2). When N is large,

$$c_+(X_1 - 2X_2)\frac{(X_1 - 2X_2 - 1)}{N} = Nc_+(\frac{X_1}{N} - 2\frac{X_2}{N})(\frac{X_1}{N} - 2\frac{X_2}{N} - \frac{1}{N})$$

$$\sim Nc_+(\frac{X_1}{N} - 2\frac{X_2}{N})^2 = N\beta(\frac{X}{N}),$$

where

$$\beta(\bar{x}) = c_+(\bar{x}_1 - 2\bar{x}_2)^2.$$

We will use this last expression in what follows. The related vector field (12.3) is then

$$
\begin{aligned}
F(\bar{x}) &= \sum_l l\beta_l(\bar{x}) \\
&= \begin{pmatrix} -1 \\ 0 \end{pmatrix} \nu\bar{x}_1 + \begin{pmatrix} 0 \\ 1 \end{pmatrix} c_+(\bar{x}_1 - 2\bar{x}_2)^2 + \begin{pmatrix} 0 \\ -1 \end{pmatrix} c_-\bar{x}_2 \\
&\quad + \sum_{n=1}^{\infty} \begin{pmatrix} n \\ 0 \end{pmatrix} p(n)\alpha(\bar{x}_2).
\end{aligned}
$$

The approximating o.d.e. (12.6) is given by the differential system

$$
\frac{d\bar{x}_1}{dt} = -\nu\bar{x}_1 + \left(\sum_{n\geq 1} np(n)\right)\alpha(\bar{x}_2) = -\nu\bar{x}_1 + b\alpha(\bar{x}_2), \tag{12.20}
$$

where b is the mean burst size, and

$$
\frac{d\bar{x}_2}{dt} = c_+(\bar{x}_1 - 2\bar{x}_2)^2 - c_-\bar{x}_2, \tag{12.21}
$$

with

$$
\bar{x}_1 - 2\bar{x}_2 \geq 0,
$$

from construction. The Jacobian $K = DF(\bar{x})$ is

$$
K = \begin{pmatrix} -\nu & b\frac{d\alpha(\bar{x}_2)}{d\bar{x}_2} \\ 2c_+(\bar{x}_1 - 2\bar{x}_2) & -4c_+(\bar{x}_1 - 2\bar{x}_2) - c_- \end{pmatrix}.
$$

The equilibria of the system given by (12.20) and (12.21) solve the system of equations

$$
\begin{aligned}
0 &= -\nu\bar{x}_1 + b\alpha(\bar{x}_2) \\
0 &= c_+(\bar{x}_1 - 2\bar{x}_2)^2 - c_-\bar{x}_2.
\end{aligned}
$$

Any equilibrium point thus satisfies the equation

$$
c_-\bar{x}_2 = c_+\left(\frac{b\alpha(\bar{x}_2)}{\nu} - 2\bar{x}_2\right)^2.
$$

Consider first the existence and uniqueness of the equilibrium. The derivative of the second term of the above equation is negative:

$$
2c_+\left(\frac{b\alpha(\bar{x}_2)}{\nu} - 2\bar{x}_2\right)\left(\frac{b\frac{d\alpha(\bar{x}_2)}{d\bar{x}_2}}{\nu} - 2\right) < 0,
$$

since α is strictly decreasing by assumption, and $\bar{x}_1 - 2\bar{x}_2 \geq 0$. Let

$$\bar{x}_* = (\bar{x}_{*1}, \bar{x}_{*2})$$

be the unique critical point. One checks then that the Jacobian K has a negative trace and a positive determinant, and hence that both eigenvalues of K have negative real parts, proving that $\bar{x}_*$ is asymptotically stable. The reader can check that condition (B.9) of theorem B.2.4 is satisfied so that the orbits of the Lyapunov equation (12.12) converge to a limiting covariance matrix Σ that solves (12.14).

The authors of [173] studied the effect of negative feedback loops using the gaussian approximation by looking at the covariance matrix as given by formulas (12.15), (12.16) and (12.17). A direct computation shows that

$$G(\bar{x}_*) = \begin{pmatrix} b(b+1)\alpha(\bar{x}_{*2}) + \nu\bar{x}_{*1} & 0 \\ 0 & c_+(\bar{x}_{*1} - 2\bar{x}_{*2})^2 + c_-\bar{x}_{*2} \end{pmatrix},$$

so that

$$\nu_{11} = -\frac{b(b+1)\alpha(\bar{x}_{*2}) + \nu\bar{x}_{*1}}{2K_{11}} \quad \text{and} \quad \nu_{22} = -\frac{c_+(\bar{x}_{*1} - 2\bar{x}_{*2})^2 + c_-\bar{x}_{*2}}{2K_{22}}.$$

Let ρ be the **negative feedback strength**

$$\rho = \frac{K_{12}}{K_{11}} = \frac{-\frac{bd\alpha(\bar{x}_{*2})}{d\bar{x}_2}}{\nu}. \tag{12.22}$$

Figure 12.6 provides an idea of the effect of negative feedback loops on noise properties, within the linear noise approximation framework. The negative feedback loop ($\rho = 100$, left panel) can reduce the variances and changes noise directions (compare with the right panel). The interested reader can consult [173] for more details. Figure 12.7 shows, however, that this effect is only valid for small enough negative feedback strength: when ρ is larger than a threshold value, the variance of the number of proteins is an increasing function of ρ. The authors of [113] considered a RNA-protein network with arbitrary negative feedback loops. They provide an interesting approach based on information theory to show the existence of fundamental limits on the suppression of molecular fluctuations. Statistical inference questions were considered in a similar setting in [25].

Negative feedback loops can also increase the frequency of noise; see [159] and [8]. These authors focus on a normalised auto-correlation function $\Phi(\tau)$, which is defined for species i as

$$\Phi_i(\tau) = \frac{\mathbb{E}(X_i(t)X_i(t+\tau))}{\mathbb{E}(X_i(t)^2)},$$

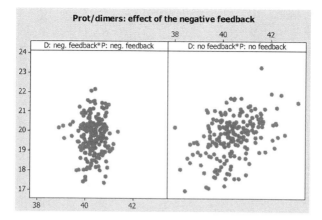

FIGURE 12.6: Effect of the negative feedback loop on noise. Left panel: strong negative feedback with $\rho = 100$. Right panel: no feedback $\rho = 0$. These plots are based on samples of size 200. Negative regulation leads to smaller variances and to changes in noise direction.

for large t. They defined $\tau_{i,1/2}$ as the time lag τ for which $\Phi_i(\tau_{i,1/2}) = 1/2$. The **noise frequency range** F_i is then defined by $F_i = \tau_{i,1/2}^{-1}$. They showed in a simple situation that F_i is larger for negatively auto-regulated genes, and argue that this might be useful for noise filtering. The authors of [8] also provide experiments which illustrate the effect of network topology on noise frequencies.

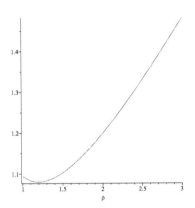

FIGURE 12.7: Variance of the number of proteins X_1 versus ρ. The variance decreases when ρ is smaller than a threshold value. However, for large enough ρ, the variance is an increasing function of ρ.

Chapter 13

Mass action kinetics

Section 12.1 focuses on laws of large numbers for reaction networks involving transitions of the form $x \to x + l$, where $x \in \mathbb{N}^M$ and $l \in \mathbb{Z}^M$, of rates $q_{x\,x+l} = N\beta_l(x/N)$, for a large parameter N. We here consider the special case where the rate functions are defined using the mass action principle, assuming well-mixed reactors of macroscopic proportions. Biological cells are neither well-mixed nor macroscopic; see, e.g., the discussion in [75]. Models based on mass action principles are, however, useful as first approximations where precise mathematical results can be obtained, which help understanding complex systems. For example, [5] showed that the steady state distributions associated with stochastic mass action dynamics are often of product form and are strongly related mathematically to the equilibrium points of the associated deterministic versions. They also extend these results to Markov processes based on Michaelis Menten transition rates, shedding light, e.g., on the results described in section 4.1 for metabolic pathways. A beautiful mathematical theory has been developed for deterministic mass action kinetics by [90], [89], [48], [49], [50] and [51].

Adopting the setting of sections 3.1 and 12.1, we consider a set of species $\mathcal{S} = \{S_1, \cdots, S_M\}$ and a family of reaction channels $\mathcal{R}$, given by the integer valued vectors $l \in \mathbb{Z}^M$. We adopt the notations of the standard literature (see, e.g., [5]) and rewrite the vectors l as

$$l = \nu'^l - \nu^l,$$

where $\nu^l \in \mathbb{N}^M$ and $\nu'^l \in \mathbb{N}^M$ have nonnegative integer valued components, and describe the number of molecules of each species consumed and created during the reaction associated with l. Let

$$X(t) = (X_1(t), \cdots, X_M(t)) \in \mathbb{N}^M$$

be the random vector giving the abundances of the various species at time t. $X(t)$, $t \geq 0$ is a Markov chain of transitions

$$x \longrightarrow x + l = (x_1 + \nu_1'^l - \nu_1^l, \cdots, x_M + \nu_M'^l - \nu_M^l),$$

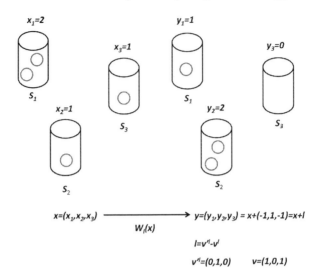

FIGURE 13.1: During a small time interval $(t, t+h)$, the system jumps from $X(t) = x$ to $X(t + h) = y = x + l$, where $l = (-1, 1, -1) = \nu'' - \nu'$, meaning that this reaction consumes one molecule of type S_1 and one molecule of type S_3 to produce one molecule of type S_2. The reaction rate is given by (13.1).

when $x = (x_1, \cdots, x_M)$. One can also rewrite this reaction as

$$\nu^l \to \nu'^l$$

to indicate that the complex ν^l is converted into ν'^l. First-order reaction networks are obtained when $\nu_i^l \in \{0, 1\}$, $i = 1, \cdots, M$. The set $\mathcal{C}$ of chemical complexes associated with $\mathcal{S}$ and $\mathcal{R}$ is $\mathcal{C} = \cup_l \{\nu^l, \nu'^l\}$, that is, $\mathcal{C}$ is the set of all the possible inputs and outputs. The set of reactions can then be described using directed edges by writing $\mathcal{E} = \{(\nu^l \to \nu'^l); \ l \in \mathcal{R}\}$. This defines a **directed graph** $\mathcal{G} = (\mathcal{C}, \mathcal{E})$ of node set $\mathcal{C}$ and of edge set $\mathcal{E}$. Let $p = |\mathcal{C}|$ and $r := |\mathcal{E}|$. A reaction network of this sort is said to be **weakly reversible** when, for each directed edge $(\nu \to \nu') \in \mathcal{E}$, there is a sequence of complexes $\nu_k \in \mathcal{C}$, $k = 1, \cdots, m - 1$ such that $(\nu' \to \nu_1) \in \mathcal{E}, \cdots, (\nu_k \to \nu_{k+1}) \in \mathcal{E}, \cdots, (\nu_m \to \nu) \in \mathcal{E}$. We adopt the notations and definitions of [49] and [172]: a complex $\nu \in \mathcal{C}$ is said to be directly linked to a complex ν', denoted by $\nu \leftrightarrow \nu'$, if either $\nu \to \nu'$ or $\nu' \to \nu$. A complex ν is said to be linked to a complex ν', denoted by $\nu \sim \nu'$, if either $\nu = \nu'$ or one can find a sequence of complexes $\nu_1, \cdots, \nu_k$ such that $\nu \leftrightarrow \nu_2 \leftrightarrow \cdots \leftrightarrow \nu_k = \nu'$. The relation $\sim$ is an equivalence relation, and the related equivalence classes are called **linkage classes**.

The propensity functions (see section 3.1) associated with mass action systems have the generic form, for $l = \nu'^l - \nu^l$,

$$W_l(x) = \kappa_l \prod_{i=1}^{M} \nu_i^l! \binom{x_i}{\nu_i^l} = \kappa_l \prod_{i=1}^{M} \frac{x_i!}{(x_i - \nu_i^l)!}, \tag{13.1}$$

when $\nu_i^l \le x_i$ for $i = 1, \cdots, M$, and is zero otherwise, for positive constants κ_l. $W_l(x)$ reflects the various possible subsets of molecules of type i, of size ν_i^l that can be consumed during reaction l. This uniform sampling scheme is valid when the particles move randomly and uniformly in the medium. The constants κ_l model the probability that such molecules meet in a volume element. Assuming the related Markov chain irreducible on $\mathbb{N}^M$, the associated steady state distribution π must satisfy the identity (see (2.7))

$$\pi(x) \sum_l W_l(x) = \sum_l \pi(x + \nu^l - \nu'^l) W_l(x + \nu^l - \nu'^l). \tag{13.2}$$

This kind of network dynamics was studied by [102], [187] and [158], among others, and more recently by [5]. The literature considers the problem of finding conditions under which π has a product form (see section 4.1 to see the biological implications of product form distributions).

13.1 Deterministic mass action kinetics and the deficiency zero theorem*

The deterministic version of these stochastic systems is obtained by proceeding as in section 12.1: one rescales the constants κ_l by setting

$$\kappa_l = \frac{\hat{\kappa}_l}{V^{|\nu^l|}},$$

where $|\nu^l| = \sum_{i=1}^{M} \nu_i^l$ is the number of molecules which are consumed during reaction l, and where V is the the system volume, which is assumed to be large. Then, following [5],

$$
\begin{aligned}
W_l(x) &= \hat{\kappa}_l V \frac{1}{V^{|\nu^l|}} \prod_{i=1}^{M} \frac{x_i!}{(x_i - \nu_i^l)!} \\
&= \hat{\kappa}_l V \prod_{i=1}^{M} \frac{x_i(x_i - 1) \cdots (x_i - \nu_i^l + 1)}{V^{\nu_i^l}} \\
&\sim V \hat{\kappa}_l \prod_{i=1}^{M} \left(\frac{x_i}{V}\right)^{\nu_i^l},
\end{aligned}
$$

when V is large, so that the propensity is such that

$$
W_l(x) \sim V \beta_l\left(\frac{x}{V}\right),
$$

where

$$
\beta_l(c) = \hat{\kappa}_l \prod_{i=1}^{M} c_i^{\nu_i^l}.
$$

We use here the notation c instead of $\bar{x}$ to denote concentrations. Proceeding as in section 12.1, one can consider the o.d.e. associated with the vector field

$$
F(c) = \sum_l l \beta_l(c) = \sum_l \hat{\kappa}_l \prod_{i=1}^{M} c_i^{\nu_{il}} (\nu'^l - \nu^l), \tag{13.3}
$$

which is the so-called **deterministic mass action kinetics**

$$
\frac{d\bar{X}(t)}{dt} = F(\bar{X}(t)). \tag{13.4}
$$

Noticing that the above vector field is a linear combination of the vectors l, one naturally defines the **stoichiometric subspace** $\mathcal{T}$ as the span of the vectors $l = \nu'^l - \nu^l$. For $x \in \mathbb{N}^M$, $x + \mathcal{T}$ and $(x + \mathcal{T}) \cap \mathbb{R}_+^M$ are the stoichiometric compatibility classes and **positive stoichiometric compatibility classes** associated with x. The **deficiency** of a reaction network of this sort is the number δ defined by

$$
\delta = \sharp \text{ complexes} - \sharp \text{ linkage classes} - \dim(\mathcal{T}).
$$

The following is the famous Feinberg theorem [49]:

Theorem 13.1.1 (Zero deficiency theorem) *Consider a weakly reversible mass action system of the form (13.4) with F given by (13.3). Suppose that $\delta = 0$. For each given positive compatibility class, there is exactly one equilibrium c^* with $F(c^*) = 0$ which is locally asymptotically stable relative to its compatibility class.*

Set

$$c^\nu = \prod_{i=1}^{M} c_i^{\nu_i}.$$

The reaction network is **complex balanced** when the following identity holds:

$$\sum_{l:\ \nu'^l = \nu} \hat{\kappa}_l c^{\nu^l} = \sum_{l:\ \nu^l = \nu} \hat{\kappa}_l c^{\nu^l}, \ \forall \nu, \tag{13.5}$$

for some $c > 0$; see, e.g., [48], [49] or [75]. One can prove the following result (see, e.g., [90] and [49], Proposition 5.3), which can be used in the stochastic case [5]. In what follows, $\ln(c)$ is the vector obtained by taking the logarithm of the components of $c \in \mathbb{R}_+^M$.

Theorem 13.1.2 *Suppose that there is a $c^* \in \mathbb{R}_+^M$ satisfying (13.5). Then the network is weakly reversible. Moreover, the following are equivalent:*

- $c \in \mathbb{R}_+^M$ *is such that $F(c) = 0$.*

- *(13.5) holds.*

- $\langle F(c), \ln(c) - \ln(c^*) \rangle \le 0$.

- $\ln(c) - \ln(c^*) \in \mathcal{T}^\perp$.

The above theorem is useful in finding the equilibria and to prove the convergence of the trajectories of (13.4). For example, the last assertion shows that $\ln(c)$ is in a coset of the orthogonal complement of the stoichiometric subspace $\mathcal{T}^\perp$. The next result is also useful in this setting:

Theorem 13.1.3 *Assume that the reaction network has zero deficiency. There exists $c \in \mathbb{R}_+^M$ such that the reaction network is complex balanced if and only if the network is weakly reversible.*

The proofs of theorems 13.1.1, 13.1.2 and 13.1.3 can be found in the works of [90] and [49], which make strong use of linear algebra. We show in what follows how one can get information on these results using classical Markov chain theory. We use the framework of section 2.2: when the network is complex balanced for some positive c, (13.5) can be recast as (2.7)

$$\sum_{l:\ \nu'^l = \nu} \mu(\nu^l) q_{\nu^l \nu} = \mu(\nu) \sum_{l:\ \nu^l = \nu} q_{\nu \nu'^l}, \tag{13.6}$$

where we set $\mu(\nu) = c^\nu$, and where the generator matrix Q is such that

$$q_{\nu \nu'} = \hat{\kappa}_l, \ l = \nu' - \nu \in \mathcal{R},$$

which is equivalent to $\mu Q = 0$. We thus look for an invariant measure μ_c for the generator Q having the special form $\mu_c(\nu) = c^\nu$, $\forall \nu \in \mathcal{C}$.

Assume that there is a single linkage class. When the reaction network is weakly reversible, the generator Q is irreducible, and there is thus a unique invariant probability measure π_κ which is given by the matrix tree theorem 2.2.4. Every invariant measure μ is then a scalar multiple of π_κ. When the network is not weakly reversible, the invariant measures μ are convex combinations of the extremal invariant measures associated with the closed irreducible subgraphs; see remark 2.2.2. One then treats these components individually since they are irreducible.

Assume in what follows that the network is weakly reversible, with a single linkage class. Let $c \in \mathbb{R}_+^M$ be such that (13.5) or (13.6) holds: there is a λ_c with

$$c^\nu = \exp(\langle \ln(c), \nu \rangle) = \lambda_c \pi_\kappa(\nu), \ \forall \nu \in \mathcal{C},$$

or, taking the logarithm on both sides,

$$\langle \ln(c), \nu \rangle = \ln(\lambda_c) + \ln(\pi_\kappa(\nu)), \ \forall \nu \in \mathcal{C}.$$

Let $[\nu]$ be the (M, p) matrix containing the complexes $\nu \in \mathcal{C}$. Then, $\ln(c)$ solves the linear equation

$$[\nu]^T \ln(c) = \ln(\lambda_c)\mathbf{1} + \ln(\pi_\kappa), \tag{13.7}$$

where $\mathbf{1}$ is the constant vector composed of ones. Furthermore, let c^* be such that (13.5) holds. Then, using the same arguments,

$$\langle \nu, \ln(c) - \ln(c^*) \rangle = (\ln(\lambda_c) - \ln(\lambda_{c^*}))\mathbf{1},$$

so that the scalar product $\langle \nu, \ln(c) - \ln(c^*) \rangle$ is independent of ν. For any pair ν, ν' of $\mathcal{C}$, one obtains that

$$\langle \nu' - \nu, \ln(c) - \ln(c^*) \rangle = 0.$$

Hence, $\ln(c) - \ln(c^*)$ is in the orthogonal complement of the span of the differences $\nu' - \nu$, where ν and ν' both belong to $\mathcal{C}$. Weak reversibility implies that the latter is the stoichiometric subspace $\mathcal{T}$: for any pair of complexes ν and ν', there is a sequence of complexes $\nu_k \in \mathcal{C}$, $k = 1, \cdots, m$ such that $(\nu \to \nu_1) \in \mathcal{E}, \cdots, (\nu_m \to \nu') \in \mathcal{E}$. Hence, $\nu' - \nu = \sum_{k=1}^{m+1}(\nu_k - \nu_{k-1}) \in \mathcal{T}$, where we set $\nu_0 = \nu$ and $\nu_{m+1} = \nu'$. We thus have proven that

$$\ln(c) - \ln(c^*) \in \mathcal{T}^\perp,$$

as claimed in theorem 13.1.2.

We next provide some ideas to better understand the notion of deficiency using the framework of [112]. Let D be the **incidence matrix** of the complex graph $\mathcal{G} = (\mathcal{C}, \mathcal{E})$, with $d_{\nu,l} = 1$ when $\nu^{\prime l} = \nu$, $d_{\nu,l} = -1$ when $\nu^l = \nu$, and with $d_{\nu,l} = 0$ otherwise. The following lemma of algebraic graph theory can be found in [18]:

Lemma 13.1.4

$$\text{rank}(D) = p - \sharp linkage\ classes,$$

$$\dim(\text{Ker}(D)) = r - p + \sharp linkage\ classes.$$

This can be seen as follows: $\text{Ker}(D^T)$ is the space of functions defined on $\mathcal{C}$ which are constant on each component, and is thus a linear subspace of dimension $\sharp$ linkage classes. The rank-nullity theorem then shows that

$$\text{rank}(D) = \text{rank}(D^T) = p - \sharp \text{linkage classes}.$$

Hence,

$$\dim(\text{Ker}(D)) = r - p + \sharp \text{linkage classes}.$$

Let $[l]$ denote the (p, r) stoichiometric matrix containing the reaction vectors $l \in \mathcal{R}$, with $\text{rank}([l]) = \dim(\mathcal{T})$, and,

$$[l] = [\nu]D. \tag{13.8}$$

Let $\beta(c) = (\beta_l(c))_l$ be the vector containing the transition rates

$$\beta_l(c) = \hat{\kappa}_l c^{\nu^l}.$$

The above definitions show that

$$F(c) = [l]\beta(c) = [\nu]D\beta(c),$$

and that (13.5) is equivalent to $D\beta(c) = 0$. The first natural observation is that for reaction networks having zero deficiency,

$$F(c) = 0 \text{ if and only if } D\beta(c) = 0.$$

This can be seen from the dimension formula

$$\dim(\text{Ker}([l])) = \dim(\text{Ker}(D)) + \dim(\text{Ker}([\nu]) \cap \text{Im}(D)).$$

The hypothesis $\delta = -\dim(\mathcal{T}) + p - \sharp$ linkage classes $= 0$ gives

$$\dim(\text{Ker}([l])) = r - \text{rank}([l]) = r - \dim(\mathcal{T}) = r - p + \sharp \text{ linkage classes},$$

so that, from lemma 13.1.4, $\dim(\text{Ker}([l])) = \dim(\text{Ker}(D))$ as required.

Example 13.1.5 [First-order reaction networks] Section 3.2 focuses on first-order reaction networks, that is, on networks where $\mathcal{C} \subset \mathcal{S} \cup \{\emptyset\}$. Each reaction is of the form $(S_i \to S_j)$, $(\emptyset \to S_i)$ or $(S_i \to \emptyset)$, where we notice that $\emptyset$ can be considered as a complex when there is a source or if degradation occurs. Each complex ν is then a unit basis vector e_i or the zero vector when the complex is $\emptyset$. When the reaction network is closed, that is, when $\mathcal{C} = \mathcal{S}$, $[\nu] = I_M$ where I_M is the identity matrix, so that $[l] = D$. Hence $\dim(\mathcal{T}) = \text{rank}([l]) = \text{rank}(D) = p - \sharp$linkage classes, so that closed first-order reaction networks have zero deficiency. One can proceed in a similar way to check that open first-order reaction networks also have zero deficiency. The reader can notice that the related mass action kinetics (13.4) corresponds to the o.d.e. (3.1); see remark 3.3.3.

13.2 Stochastic mass action kinetics

The Markov chain associated with the transition rates (13.1) evolves in the countable state space $\mathbb{N}^M$, and the general problem of finding invariant probability measures satisfying (13.2) represents in general a formidable task. Moreover, such chains are not necessarily irreducible. In the latter case, one must consider the set of closed and irreducible components of the state space and look for the extremal invariant probability measures; see remark 2.2.2. The following result can be found in [5]. Interestingly, the existence of an invariant measure is related to the existence of some $c \in \mathbb{R}_+^M$ ensuring that the network is complex balanced.

Theorem 13.2.1 *Assume that the reaction network is complex balanced for some $c^* \in \mathbb{R}_+^M$ which solves $F(c^*) = 0$. Then the associated Markov chain has an invariant measure π of Poisson type with*

$$\pi(x) = \prod_{i=1}^{M} \frac{c_i^{x_i}}{x_i!} e^{-c_i},$$

where the vector $c = (c_i)$ is an equilibrium of the deterministic system given by (13.4) and (13.3). If the chain is irreducible, then π is the unique steady state distribution. If the chain is reducible, each extremal invariant probability measure π_A (see remark 2.2.2) associated with some closed and irreducible *subset A is of the form*

$$\pi_A(x) = \frac{1}{Z_A} \prod_{i=1}^{M} \frac{c_i^{x_i}}{x_i!}, \quad x \in A,$$

where Z_A is a normalisation constant, and where $c = (c_i)$ is an equilibrium value of the differential system defined by (13.4) and (13.3).

The Poisson distribution is an invariant measure when (13.2) holds; plugging the Poisson distribution in the latter and using mass action propensities one obtains the relation

$$\sum_l \kappa_l \prod_i \frac{1}{(x_i - \nu_i^l)!} = \sum_l \kappa_l \prod_i \frac{c_i^{\nu_i^l - \nu_i'^l}}{(x_i - \nu_i'^l)!}.$$

Equivalently, one can write

$$\sum_\nu \prod_i \frac{1}{(x_i - \nu_i)!} \sum_{l:\, \nu^l = \nu} \kappa_l = \sum_\nu \prod_i \frac{1}{(x_i - \nu_i)!} \sum_{l:\, \nu'^l = \nu} \kappa_l \prod_i c_i^{\nu_i^l - \nu_i},$$

which is satisfied when the following identities hold $\forall \nu$:

$$\prod_i c_i^{\nu_i} \sum_{l:\, \nu^l = \nu} \kappa_l = \sum_{l:\, \nu'^l = \nu} \kappa_l \prod_i c_i^{\nu_i^l},$$

which is (13.5) when $\hat{\kappa}_l = \kappa_l$.

Example 13.2.2 [Enzymatic kinetics] Enzymatic reactions are ubiquitous in biochemical reaction networks and are instrumental for cellular processing. Examples 2.2.8 and 2.4.2 propose to model such reactions using Markov chains. Section 4.1 focuses on reaction networks which are built on interacting enzymatic kinetics and explains why product-form steady state distributions might be relevant for adaptation. We consider here more general networks of conversion type where substrate S_i can be transformed into substrates S_j, through the action of enzymes E. These reactions are represented by the relations

$$S_i + E \underset{\kappa_-^{ij}}{\overset{\kappa_+^{ij}}{\longleftrightarrow}} (S_i - E - S_j) \underset{\hat{\kappa}_-^{ij}}{\overset{\hat{\kappa}_+^{ij}}{\longleftrightarrow}} S_j + E. \tag{13.9}$$

We suppose here that the enzyme E can be produced or degraded according to the relation

$$\emptyset \underset{\nu}{\overset{\mu}{\longleftrightarrow}} E. \tag{13.10}$$

The first relation can be represented by a graph $\mathcal{G}^0$ of node set $\{S_i + E,\ i =$

$1, \cdots, M\}$. There is an edge between the complexes $S_i + E$ and $S_j + E$ when S_i can be converted into S_j through the action of the enzyme E and vice versa. The set of such (nonoriented) edges will be denoted by $\mathcal{E}^0$. We assume here that the graph $\mathcal{G}^0$ is connected, so that the corresponding complex graph has a single linkage class. The second component of the global complex graph which encompasses also the second relation has two linkage classes. The related set of species is $\{S_1, \cdots, S_M\} \cup \{E\} \cup \{S_i - E - S_j; \ (ij) \in \mathcal{E}^0\}$, and the set of complexes is

$$\mathcal{C} = \{S_i + E; \ S_i \in \mathcal{S}\} \cup \{\emptyset\} \cup \{E\} \cup \{S_i - E - S_j; \ (ij) \in \mathcal{E}^0\}.$$

This reaction network has

$$|\mathcal{C}| = M + |\mathcal{E}^0| + 2$$

complexes and two linkage classes. Each complex $S_i + E$ is represented by the sum of the corresponding unit vectors $e_i + e_{M+1}$, where e_{M+1} is the standard basis vector associated with the enzyme E. Likewise, each complex $S_i - E - S_j$ is represented by a basis vector e_{ij} (all of these various unit basis vectors are linearly independent). Reactions of the form

$$S_i + E \underset{\kappa_-^{ij}}{\overset{\kappa_+^{ij}}{\longleftrightarrow}} (S_i - E - S_j),$$

are thus associated with reaction vectors $l = e_{ij} - e_i - e_{M+1}$. Considering only the first set of relations, which is associated with the first linkage class, we observe that the related stoichiometric matrix is the incidence matrix of the graph $\mathcal{G}^0$. The dimension of the associated stoichiometric subspace is $M + |\mathcal{E}^0| - 1$; see lemma 13.1.4. Taking into account the second relation (13.10), one obtains that

$$\dim(\mathcal{T}) = (M + |\mathcal{E}^0| - 1) + 1 = M + |\mathcal{E}^0|,$$

so that this reaction network has zero deficiency. This network is also weakly reversible since the graph $\mathcal{G}^0$ was assumed to be connected, and we can thus find a positive c so that the network is complex balanced.

The stochastic mass action dynamics is not irreducible: Let $X_i(t)$ and $X_{ij}(t)$, $(ij) \in \mathcal{E}^0$ denote the number of type i species and of $S_i - E - S_j$ complexes present in the system at time t. Assume that $\sum_{i=1}^{M} X_i(0) + \sum_{(i,j) \in \mathcal{E}^0} X_{ij}(0) = N$ for some number $N > 0$. Let $X_E(t)$ denote the number of enzymes at time t. Relations (13.9) model conversions of substrate molecules, so that the number of substrate molecules is preserved with

$\sum_{i=1}^{M} X_i(t) + \sum_{(i,j) \in \mathcal{E}^0} X_{ij}(t) \equiv N$, $\forall t \geq 0$. The process evolves then in the irreducible component

$$A_N = \{(x_1, \cdots, x_M, x_E, x_{ij}); \sum_{i=1}^{M} x_i + \sum_{(i,j) \in \mathcal{E}^0} x_{ij} = N; \ x_E \in \mathbb{N}\},$$

and theorem 13.2.1 shows that the related stationary distribution π_{A_N} is of product form

$$\pi_{A_N}(x) = \frac{c_E^{x_E}}{x_E!} e^{-c_E} \frac{\binom{N}{x_1 \cdots x_{ij} \cdots}}{Z} \prod_{i=1}^{M} c_i^{x_i} \prod_{(ij) \in \mathcal{E}^0} c_{ij}^{x_{ij}},$$

where $Z = (\sum_i c_i + \sum_{(i,j) \in \mathcal{E}^0} c_{ij})^N$, which is the product of a Poisson distribution (for the marginal law of X_E) and of a multinomial distribution involving the random variables $X_1, \cdots, X_M$ and X_{ij}, $(ij) \in \mathcal{E}^0$, which are not independent at steady state.

Example 13.2.3 [Hopf bifurcation in chemical reaction networks] The kind of reactions defined in example 13.2.2 can lead to multistationarity; see, e.g., [119], and also to Hopf bifurcation. We present here the simplest reaction network for which Hopf bifurcation appears, following the works of [188], [189] and [160], the latter giving a complete mathematical analysis. This reaction takes the form

$$A + E \xrightarrow{\kappa_1} A + A,$$
$$A + B \xrightarrow{\kappa_2} E + B,$$
$$B \xrightarrow{\kappa_3} E,$$
$$A \xrightarrow{\kappa_4} C,$$
$$C \xrightarrow{\kappa_4} B,$$

where E is the enzyme, the concentration of which is assumed to be large. The above set of relations is a mixture of enzymatic and conversion reactions. The associated mass action dynamic is

$$\frac{dc_1}{dt} = (\kappa_E - \kappa_4)c_1 - \kappa_2 c_1 c_2,$$
$$\frac{dc_2}{dt} = -\kappa_3 c_2 + \kappa_5 c_3,$$
$$\frac{dc_3}{dt} = \kappa_4 c_1 - \kappa_5 c_3,$$

where $\kappa_E = \kappa_1[E]$, and $[E]$ is the enzyme concentration. One can check that the system possess the equilibria

$$c^{(0)} = 0 \text{ and } c^{(1)} = (\frac{(\kappa_E - \kappa_4)\kappa_3}{\kappa_2 \kappa_4}, \frac{\kappa_E - \kappa_4}{\kappa_2}, \frac{(\kappa_E - \kappa_4)\kappa_3}{\kappa_2 \kappa_5}).$$

The firs one $c^{(0)}$ is stable provided $0 \leq \kappa_E < \kappa_4$, while the second one $c^{(1)}$ is stable when $\kappa_4 < \kappa_E < \kappa_3 + \kappa_4 + \kappa_5$. When κ_E crosses the threshold $\kappa_3 + \kappa_4 + \kappa_5$, the system undergoes a Hopf bifurcation where $c^{(1)}$ changes from a stable equilibrium to a stable limit cycle. The authors of [108] studied parameter estimation at bifurcation and showed that the Fisher information exhibits a singular behaviour.

13.3 Extension to more general dynamics

The results obtained for propensity functions (13.1) associated with stochastic mass action systems like

$$W_l(x) = \kappa_l \prod_{i=1}^{M} \nu_i^l! \binom{x_i}{\nu_i^l} = \kappa_l \prod_{i=1}^{M} \frac{x_i!}{(x_i - \nu_i^l)!},$$

have been extended to more general dynamics in [5]. This new class of transition rates contains Michaelis Menten reaction rates, which have been defined in section 4.1. Consider propensity functions of the form

$$W_l(x) = \kappa_l \prod_{i=1}^{M} \prod_{j=0}^{\nu_i^l - 1} \theta_i(x_i - j) \tag{13.11}$$

where one sets $\prod_{j=0}^{-1} = 0$. The functions $\theta_i : \mathbb{Z} \longrightarrow \mathbb{R}_+$ are arbitrary but must be such that $\theta_i(x) = 0$ for $x \leq 0$. Michaelis Menten type rates are obtained when

$$\theta_i(x) = \frac{\kappa_i x}{K_i + x}, \tag{13.12}$$

for positive constants κ_i and K_i; see, e.g., (4.1).

Theorem 13.3.1 *Assume that the reaction network based on rates of the form (13.11) is complex balanced for some $c \in \mathbb{R}_+^M$. Then the associated Markov chain has an invariant measure π of product form with*

$$\pi(x) = \frac{1}{Z} \prod_{i=1}^{M} \frac{c_i^{x_i}}{\prod_{j=1}^{x_i} \theta_i(j)}, \tag{13.13}$$

for a normalisation constant $Z > 0$, provided the above measure is summable. If the chain is irreducible, then (13.13) is the unique steady state distribution. If the chain is reducible, the each extremal invariant probability measure π_A (see remark 2.2.2) associated with some closed and irreducible subset A is of the form

$$\pi_A(x) = \frac{1}{Z_A} \prod_{i=1}^{M} \frac{c_i^{x_i}}{\prod_{j=1}^{x_i} \theta_i(j)}, \quad x \in A,$$

where Z_A is a normalisation constant.

We illustrate this last theorem in the framework of metabolic pathways; see section 4.1. The set of species $\mathcal{S}$ corresponds to substrate molecules, which are converted in a linear cascade through the action of enzymatic reactions (see (4.3))

$$S_i + E_i \underset{\kappa_-^i}{\overset{\kappa_+^i}{\rightleftharpoons}} (SE)_i \overset{\kappa_2^i}{\longrightarrow} S_{i+1}.$$

Assume for simplicity that the above reactions are summarised by transitions $(S_i \to S_{i+1})$, and, more generally, by transitions of the form $(S_i \to S_j)$, as considered in example 13.2.2. Let $\mathcal{G}^0$ be the related graph, of node set $\mathcal{S} \cup \{\emptyset\}$, and of edge set $\mathcal{E}^0 = \{(S_i \to S_j)\}$.

Assume for convenience that this system is of first-order, neglecting thus the full enzymatic reactions by only focusing on transitions of the form $(S_i \to S_j)$. The reaction network has thus zero deficiency; see example 13.1.5. Assume furthermore that the reaction network is weakly reversible, so that, by theorem 13.1.3, there is some positive c such that the reaction network is complex balanced. The complexes are again the unit basis vectors e_i, and the reaction vector associated with a transition $(S_i \to S_j)$ is $l = e_j - e_i$. Suppose as in section 4.1 that the reaction rates are given by the Michaelis Menten functions (13.12). Theorem 13.3.1 asserts then that the Markov chain possesses a steady state distribution of product form

$$\pi(x) = \frac{1}{Z} \prod_{i=1}^{M} \frac{c_i^{x_i}}{\prod_{j=1}^{x_i} \theta_i(j)},$$

which is, when the chain is irreducible, the unique invariant probability measure when this measure is summable. We therefore see that product form distributions appear to be quite natural in metabolic pathways (see section 4.1).

Part V

Appendix

Appendix A

Self-regulated genes

A.1 Dimerisation

A.1.1 The invariant measure

Dimerisation appears in most biochemical processes and is usually considered as a fast reaction. The aim of this section is to give mathematical statements relevant for computational purposes (see, e.g., [36], [28], [104] or [58]). Given a fixed number of proteins x, the dimerisation process is given by the reaction

$$\mathcal{M} + \mathcal{M} \xrightleftharpoons[c_-]{c_+} \mathcal{D},$$

where $\mathcal{M}$ and $\mathcal{D}$ represent monomers and dimers. Assume that the number of dimers $D(t)$ at time t is given by $D(t) = d$, so that the number of free monomers is $x - 2d$. The number of ways of creating a new dimer is given by the product $(x - 2d)(x - 2d - 1)$. Hence, assuming that each dimer can be degraded at some rate c_-, one gets the following infinitesimal transition rate:

$$P(D(t + h) = d + 1 | D(t) = d) \sim c_+ (x - 2d)(x - 2d - 1)\, h,$$

$$P(D(t + h) = d - 1 | D(t) = d) \sim c_-\, d\, h,$$

when $h \approx 0$. The related master equation is then of the form

$$
\begin{aligned}
\frac{dP_d(t)}{dt} &= c_+(x - 2(d-1))(x - 2(d-1) - 1)P_{d-1}(t) + c_-(d+1)P_{d+1}(t) \\
&\quad - (c_+(x - 2d)(x - 2d - 1) + c_- d)P_d(t),
\end{aligned}
$$

where $P_d(t) = P(D(t) = d)$. The unique stationary distribution μ^x of the process is given explicitly by

$$\mu^x(d) = \left(\frac{c_+}{c_-}\right)^d \frac{1}{(x - 2d)!\, d!} \frac{1}{Z_x}, \quad 0 \le d \le x_2, \tag{A.1}$$

where $x_2 := [x/2]$ is the integer part of x, and where

$$Z_x = \sum_{d=0}^{x_2} \left(\frac{2c_+}{c_-}\right)^d \frac{1}{(x-2d)!\, d!\, 2^d}. \tag{A.2}$$

A.1.2 Computing the moments of the invariant measure

As we will see in the next section, computation at quasi-equilibrium where dimerisation is a fast reaction requires various moments of μ^x like its expected value or its variance. The first natural approach consists in using the master equation to deduce some differential equation for these moments. Let $m_j(t) := \sum_d^{x_2} d^j P_d(t)$ be the jth moment of $D(t)$, $P_{-1}(t) = P_{x_2+1}(t) = 0$. One can consider the derivative of $m_1(t)$ to deduce a differential equation, which involves the second moment $m_2(t)$:

$$\frac{dm_1(t)}{dt} = c_+x(x-1) - (c_- + 2c_+(2x-1))m_1(t) + 4c_+m_2(t).$$

This shows that there is some difficulty in getting a simple differential equation for the first moment (this is a consequence of the quadratic nature of the transition rates). Consider the generating function

$$G(s,t) = \sum_{d=0}^{x_2} P_d(t)s^d.$$

The master equation then yields the partial differential equation

$$\frac{\partial G(s,t)}{\partial t} = c_+x(x-1)(s-1)G(s,t)$$

$$+\left((4x+2)c_+s - c_-\right)(s-1)\frac{\partial G(s,t)}{\partial s} + 4c_+s^2(s-1)\frac{\partial^2 G(s,t)}{\partial s^2},$$

which is difficult to solve. Considering the steady state and setting

$$M(s) = \lim_{t\to\infty} G(s,t) = \sum_{d=0}^{x_2} \mu^x(d)s^d,$$

the above equation yields that

$$0 = c_+x(x-1)M(s) + \left((4x+2)c_+s - c_-\right)M'(s) + 4c_+s^2M''(s). \tag{A.3}$$

This equation is formally solved by a linear combination of the two confluent hypergeometric functions (see [36]) as

$$2^{x-1}\left(\frac{c_+}{c_-}\right)^{\frac{x-1}{2}} s^{\frac{x-1}{2}} {}_1F_1\left(\frac{1-x}{2}, \frac{3}{2}, -\frac{c_-}{4c_+s}\right),$$

and

$$2^x \left(\frac{c_+}{c_-}\right)^{\frac{x}{2}} s^{\frac{x}{2}} {}_1F_1\left(\frac{-x}{2}, \frac{1}{2}, -\frac{c_-}{4c_+ s}\right).$$

$M(s)$ being a polynomial of degree x_2 with $M(1) = 1$, one of the factors of the linear combination vanishes, and the other is a normalising constant, so that

$$M(s) = \begin{cases} s^{x_2} \dfrac{{}_1F_1\left(-x_2, \frac{3}{2}, -\frac{c_-}{4c_+ s}\right)}{{}_1F_1\left(-x_2, \frac{3}{2}, -\frac{c_-}{4c_+}\right)}, & \text{if } x \text{ is odd}, \\[4ex] s^{x_2} \dfrac{{}_1F_1\left(-x_2, \frac{1}{2}, -\frac{c_-}{4c_+ s}\right)}{{}_1F_1\left(-x_2, \frac{1}{2}, -\frac{c_-}{4c_+}\right)}, & \text{if } x \text{ is even}. \end{cases}$$

The above representation gives a theoretical way of computing the invariant measure as

$$\mu^x(d) = \frac{M^{(d)}(0)}{d!}, \qquad 0 \le d \le x_2,$$

and the mean number of dimers in the steady state is given by

$$\mathbb{E}_x = M'(1).$$

Numerical computation based on this last formula is problematic, even for x relatively small, say 1000. The reader can consult [58], where iterative algorithms are provided to evaluate the moments of μ^x.

A.2 Transcription with fast dimerisation

The model is similar to that given in chapter 1, where protein monomers fist form dimers before binding to the promoter region. We assume here that dimerisation is a fast process. The set of chemical reactions is described by the relation

$$\mathcal{M} \xrightarrow{\nu} \emptyset, \quad \emptyset \xrightarrow{\mu_l} \mathcal{M}, \ l \in \{0, 1\}, \quad \mathcal{O}_0 + \mathcal{D} \underset{\kappa}{\overset{g}{\longleftrightarrow}} \mathcal{O}_1, \quad \mathcal{M} + \mathcal{M} \underset{\beta_-^\varepsilon}{\overset{\beta_+^\varepsilon}{\longleftrightarrow}} \mathcal{D},$$

where $\mathcal{D}$ represent dimers, g is function of the number of dimers, and the rates β_-^ε and β_+^ε involve a small number $\varepsilon > 0$ modelling the speed of dimerization. The number $X^\varepsilon(t)$ of proteins $\mathcal{P}$ present at time t is related to the number of dimers as $0 \le 2D^\varepsilon(t) \le X^\varepsilon(t)$, and the number of free monomers is such that $\mathcal{M} + 2\mathcal{D} = \mathcal{P}$. Let $Y^\varepsilon(t) = 0, 1$ be the state of the promoter (OFF/ON) at time

t. We illustrate in what follows the notion of quasi-equilibrium in this example.

The running process is a Markov chain

$$\eta^\varepsilon(t) = (X^\varepsilon(t), Y^\varepsilon(t), D^\varepsilon(t)) \in \mathbb{N} \text{ x } \{0, 1\} \text{ x } \mathbb{N},$$

with $0 \le 2D^\varepsilon(t) \le X^\varepsilon(t)$, of generator Q^ε. The associated transition rates are given in Table A.1 below.

TABLE A.1: The different types of interactions involved in the self-regulated gene

Name	transition	rate
Production (ON)	$(x, 1, d) \longrightarrow (x + 1, 1, d)$	μ_1
Production (OFF)	$(x, 0, d) \longrightarrow (x + 1, 0, d)$	μ_0
Degradation	$(x, y, d) \longrightarrow (x - 1, y, d)$	νx
Conversion (OFF/ON)	$(x, 0, d) \longrightarrow (x, 1, d)$	$g(d)$
Conversion (ON/OFF)	$(x, 1, d) \longrightarrow (x, 0, d)$	κ
Production (dimers)	$(x, y, d) \longrightarrow (x, y, d + 1)$	$c_+(x - 2d)(x - 2d - 1)/\varepsilon$
Degradation (dimers)	$(x, y, d) \longrightarrow (x, y, d - 1)$	c_-/ε

The dimerisation process $D^\varepsilon(t)$ is defined by the rates provided in Table A.2.

TABLE A.2: Reaction rates associated with the fast dimerisation process.

Name	transition	rate
Production (dimers)	$(x, y, d) \longrightarrow (x, y, d + 1)$	$c_+(x - 2d)(x - 2d - 1)/\varepsilon$
Degradation (dimers)	$(x, y, d) \longrightarrow (x, y, d - 1)$	c_-/ε

We use the setting of section 2.4 as follows: let

$$\mathcal{E}_s = \{(x, y); \ 0 \le x \le M; \ y = 0, \ 1\},$$

and, for $k = (x, y) \in \mathcal{E}_s$,

$$E_k = \{(x, y, d); \ 0 \le 2d \le x\}.$$

Notice that we have truncated the process by imposing that the number of proteins is bounded by M. This can be done by modifying the generator slightly.

One recovers the infinite case when M is large (see [58] for some mathematical issues on this topic).

For $k = (x, y) \in \mathcal{E}_s$, the generator A^k defined in section 2.4 is simply given by the reaction rate $c_+(x - 2d)(x - 2d - 1)$ for the transition $(x, y, d) \rightarrow (x, y, d+1)$, and by the rate $c_- d$ for the reaction $(x, y, d) \rightarrow (x, y, d-1)$. Hence, the steady state measure $\sigma^{(x,y)}$ defined in section 2.4 is simply the invariant probability measure μ^x of section A.1.1.

TABLE A.3: The slow reaction rates defining the generator B.

Name	transition	rate
Production (ON)	$(x, 1, d) \longrightarrow (x + 1, 1, d)$	μ_1
Production (OFF)	$(x, 0, d) \longrightarrow (x + 1, 0, d)$	μ_0
Degradation	$(x, y, d) \longrightarrow (x - 1, y, d)$	νx
Conversion (OFF/ON)	$(x, 0, d) \longrightarrow (x, 1, d)$	$g(d)$
Conversion (ON/OFF)	$(x, 1, d) \longrightarrow (x, 0, d)$	κ

One can then use formula (2.23) to get the rates associated with the process running at quasi-equilibrium. The only rate which depends on d corresponds to the reaction $(x, 0, d) \longrightarrow (x, 1, d)$, of rate $g(d)$. Hence, one gets the limiting rate

$$\gamma_{(x,0),(x,1)} = g(x) = \sum_{0 \le d \le [x/2]} \sigma^{(x,y)}(d) g(d), \text{ where } \sigma^{(x,y)} = \mu^x.$$

The limiting process

$$\eta(t) = (X(t), Y(t)) \in \mathbb{N} \times \{0, 1\}$$

is then defined through the transition rates provided in Table A.4.

A typical example is given by $g(D^\varepsilon(t)) = \lambda D^\varepsilon(t) + g(0)$, that is, depends linearly on the number of dimers at time t. Hence,

$$g(x) = \sum_{0 \le d \le [x/2]} \mu^x(d)(\lambda d + g(0)) = \lambda \mathbb{E}_x + g(0), \tag{A.4}$$

where we set

$$\mathbb{E}_x := \sum_{0 \le d \le [x/2]} d \mu^x(d),$$

showing the necessity of computing the first moment $\mathbb{E}_x$ of μ^x for every x when

TABLE A.4: Reaction rates associated with the self-regulated gene at quasi-equilibrium.

Name	transition	rate
Production (ON)	$(x, 1) \longrightarrow (x+1, 1)$	μ_1
Production (OFF)	$(x, 0) \longrightarrow (x+1, 0)$	μ_0
Degradation	$(x, y) \longrightarrow (x-1, y)$	νx
Conversion (OFF/ON)	$(x, 0) \longrightarrow (x, 1)$	$g(x)$
Conversion (ON/OFF)	$(x, 1) \longrightarrow (x, 0)$	κ

considering quasi-equilibrium. Efficient iterative algorithms for computing the various moments are provided in [57].

A.2.1 Inclusion of negative feedback

When the rate κ also depends on the number of dimers, that is, when $\kappa = \kappa(d)$, one can proceed in a similar way to get a process evolving at quasi-equilibrium, as described by the rates provided in Table A.5.

TABLE A.5: Reaction rates associated with the self-regulated gene at quasi-equilibrium, with possibly positive and negative feedback.

Name	transition	rate
Production (ON)	$(x, 1) \longrightarrow (x+1, 1)$	μ_1
Production (OFF)	$(x, 0) \longrightarrow (x+1, 0)$	μ_0
Degradation	$(x, y) \longrightarrow (x-1, y)$	νx
Conversion (OFF/ON)	$(x, 0) \longrightarrow (x, 1)$	$g(x)$
Conversion (ON/OFF)	$(x, 1) \longrightarrow (x, 0)$	$\kappa(x)$

A.3 Steady state distribution: the method of transfer matrices

The literature contains many examples where such modules are studied using various approximation schemes. The steady state distribution is quite often approached using highly optimised Gillespie algorithms; see, e.g., [74].

Our formula below gives the exact formula for computing the steady-state. We truncate the state space by imposing a maximal number of molecules: let Λ be the set

$$\Lambda = \{(x,y);\ 0 \leq x \leq M;\ y = 0,\ 1\}.$$

TABLE A.6: Transition rates associated with the self-regulated gene at quasi-equilibrium, in the special case where $\mu_0 = 0$.

Name	transition	rate
Production (ON)	$(x,1) \longrightarrow (x+1,1)$	μ_1
Production (OFF)	$(x,0) \longrightarrow (x+1,0)$	μ_0
Degradation	$(x,y) \longrightarrow (x-1,y)$	$\nu(x)$
Conversion (OFF/ON)	$(x,0) \longrightarrow (x,1)$	$g(x)$
Conversion (ON/OFF)	$(x,1) \longrightarrow (x,0)$	$\kappa(x)$

We assume furthermore that transitions of the form $(x,1) \longrightarrow (x+1,1)$ occur at rate $\mu_1 = \mu$ when $x \leq M-1$, and that the production rate $\mu_1 = 0$ when $x \geq M$. The degradation rate function $\nu(x)$ is assumed to be arbitrary. Table A.6 defines the transition rates of the time-continuous Markov chain associated with the self-regulated gene of reaction scheme (1.14):

$$\mathcal{M} \xrightarrow{\nu_x} \emptyset,\quad \emptyset \xrightarrow{\mu_l} \mathcal{M},\ l \in \{0,1\},\quad \mathcal{O}_0 + \mathcal{M} \underset{\kappa(x)}{\overset{g(x)}{\rightleftarrows}} \mathcal{O}_1.$$

The steady state distribution

$$\pi_x(y) = \lim_{t \to \infty} P(X(t) = x, Y(t) = y)$$

solves the equation

$$0 = \mu_y(\pi_{x-1}(y) - \pi_x(y)) + \nu(x+1)\pi_{x+1}(y) - \nu(x)\pi_x(y))$$

$$+(-1)^y(\kappa(x)\pi_x(1) - g(x)\pi_x(0)),\ y = 0,\ 1;$$

see section 1.3. We present the results of [23], [58] and [57], which give precise formulas for the steady state distribution using the method of transfer matrices.

The invariant measure $\pi_x(y)$ is related to the steady state distribution $\tilde{\pi}_x(y)$ of the associated discrete time jump chain: $\tilde{\pi}_x(y)$ is proportional to

$\pi_x(y)q_{x,y}$, where $q_{x,y}$ is the sum of the transition rates from state (x, y), see section 2.2.2. For $0 < x < M$, consider the matrices

$$Q_{x+1} = \begin{pmatrix} \frac{\nu(x+1)}{d_{x+1}} & 0 \\ 0 & \frac{\nu(x+1)}{c_{x+1}} \end{pmatrix}, \quad R_x = \begin{pmatrix} 0 & \frac{g(x)}{d_x} \\ \frac{\kappa(x)}{c_x} & 0 \end{pmatrix}$$

and

$$P_{x-1} = \begin{pmatrix} \frac{\mu_0}{d_{x-1}} & 0 \\ 0 & \frac{\mu_1}{c_{x-1}} \end{pmatrix},$$

where $c_x = \nu(x) + \mu_1 + \kappa(x)$, $x < M$, $c_M = \nu(M) + \kappa(M)$, and $d_x = \nu(x) + \mu_0 + g(x)$ for $x < M$, $d_M = \nu(M) + g(M)$. Let $\tilde{\pi}_x$ be the row vector $\tilde{\pi}_x = (\tilde{\pi}_x(0), \tilde{\pi}_x(1))$. The steady state equation shows that $\tilde{\pi}$ is such that

$$\tilde{\pi}_x = \tilde{\pi}_{x+1}Q_{x+1} + \tilde{\pi}_x R_x + \tilde{\pi}_{x-1}P_{x-1}.$$

The idea of the authors of [23] is to look for matrices α_x such that

$$\tilde{\pi}_x = \tilde{\pi}_{x+1}\alpha_x.$$

Plugging this relation into the above yields that $\tilde{\pi}_x = \tilde{\pi}_{x+1}Q_{x+1}\gamma_{x-1}$, where the matrices γ_x are defined by

$$\gamma_{x-1} = (\text{id} - R_x - \alpha_{x-1}P_{x-1})^{-1}. \tag{A.5}$$

The matrices α_n thus solve the following matrix valued continued fraction:

$$\alpha_x = Q_{x+1}(\text{id} - R_x - \alpha_{x-1}P_{x-1})^{-1}. \tag{A.6}$$

This provides an algorithm for computing exactly the steady state distribution in the general case. The authors of [23] provide sufficient conditions ensuring that the above matrices are well defined.

An explicit formula

When $\mu_0 = 0$ and $\mu_1 = \mu$, it turns out that one can solve explicitly (A.6). The solution is given by

$$\alpha_x = \frac{\nu(x+1)}{\mu} \begin{pmatrix} \frac{\kappa(x)+\mu}{d_{x+1}} & \frac{c_x}{d_{x+1}} \\ \frac{\kappa(x)}{c_{x+1}} & \frac{c_x}{c_{x+1}} \end{pmatrix}.$$

The proof is based on methods presented in [23], but here we solve explicitly (A.6). We extend the previous definitions to the boundaries as follows: set

$$\hat{R}_0 = \begin{pmatrix} 0 & 1 \\ \frac{\kappa(0)}{\kappa(0)+\mu} & 0 \end{pmatrix}, \quad Q_1 = \begin{pmatrix} \frac{\nu(1)}{d_1} & 0 \\ 0 & \frac{\nu(1)}{c_1} \end{pmatrix},$$

$$P_0 = \begin{pmatrix} 0 & 0 \\ 0 & \frac{\mu}{c_0} \end{pmatrix}, \quad \hat{R}_M = \begin{pmatrix} 0 & \frac{g(M)}{\nu(M)+g(M)} \\ \frac{\kappa(M)}{\kappa(M)+\nu(M)} & 0 \end{pmatrix},$$

$$\hat{Q}_M = \begin{pmatrix} \frac{\nu(M)}{\nu(M)+g(M)} & 0 \\ 0 & \frac{\nu(M)}{\nu(M)+\kappa(M)} \end{pmatrix}.$$

The matrices $\hat{R}_0 + P_0$ and $\hat{R}_M + \hat{Q}_M$ are stochastic. We shall see later that these matrices α_x and the inverse (A.5) are well defined; this implies that $\alpha_x = Q_{x+1}\gamma_{x-1}$. To start the induction, one needs to define α_0: this is obtained by using the invariance of $\tilde{\pi}$ at the left boundary $x = 0$, which gives $\tilde{\pi}_0 = \tilde{\pi}_0 \hat{R}_0 + \tilde{\pi}_1 Q_1$, that is, $\tilde{\pi}_0 = \tilde{\pi}_1 Q_1 (\text{id} - \hat{R}_0)^{-1}$. One gets thus the natural candidate $\alpha_0 = Q_1(\text{id} - \hat{R}_0)^{-1}$.

Lemma A.3.1 *Suppose that the matrices α_x and γ_x are well defined. Then the matrices $\theta_{x+1} = \gamma_x P_{x+1}$, $0 \le x < M - 1$, are stochastic.*

Proof: The proof proceeds by induction. When $x = 0$, we first check that $\theta_1 = \gamma_0 P_1$ is stochastic, with $\gamma_0^{-1} = \text{id} - R_1 - \alpha_0 P_0$. Let $\mathbf{1} = (1, 1)'$ be the vector having ones as components. Then $\theta_1 \mathbf{1} = \mathbf{1}$ is equivalent to $(P_1 + R_1)\mathbf{1} = \mathbf{1} - \alpha_0 P_0 \mathbf{1}$, and therefore to $0 = Q_1 \mathbf{1} - \alpha_0 P_0 \mathbf{1} = Q_1(\mathbf{1} - (\text{id} - \hat{R}_0)^{-1} P_0 \mathbf{1})$, where we use the fact that $P_1 + Q_1 + R_1$ is stochastic. But Q_1 is diagonal, and the last statement is equivalent to $(\text{id} - \hat{R}_0)\mathbf{1} = P_0 \mathbf{1}$, which holds true since $\hat{R}_0 + P_0$ is stochastic. The induction step is obtained in the same way.

Suppose that we have already obtained the sequence α_k, $k = 0, \cdots, x - 1$. Then we can obtain α_x by setting $\alpha_x = Q_{x+1}\gamma_{x-1}$. The above lemma gives that $\gamma_{x-1} P_x$ is stochastic. But, taking into account the specific form of the involved matrices, one can write

$$\gamma_{x-1} P_x = \begin{pmatrix} 0 & \frac{\mu}{c_x}\gamma_{x-1}(1,2) \\ 0 & \frac{\mu}{c_x}\gamma_{x-1}(2,2) \end{pmatrix},$$

where $\gamma_{x-1}(i,j)$ denotes the (i,j) entry of the matrix γ_{x-1}. Thus $\gamma_{x-1}(1,2) = \gamma_{x-1}(2,2) = \frac{c_x}{\mu}$. Finally, $\alpha_x = Q_{x+1}\gamma_{x-1}$ shows that $\alpha_x(1,2) = \frac{\nu(x+1)c_x}{d_{x+1}\mu}$ and $\alpha_x(2,2) = \frac{\nu(x+1)c_n}{\mu c_{x+1}}$. Let $A_{x-1} = \gamma_{x-1}^{-1}$, with

$$A_{x-1} = \begin{pmatrix} 1 & -\frac{g(x)}{d_x} - \frac{\mu \alpha_{x-1}(1,2)}{c_{x-1}} \\ -\frac{\kappa(x)}{c_x} & 1 - \frac{\mu \alpha_{x-1}(2,2)}{c_{x-1}} \end{pmatrix},$$

of determinant $|A_{x-1}|$ given by $|A_{x-1}| = \frac{\mu}{c_x}$. It follows that

$$
\begin{aligned}
\alpha_x &= \frac{c_x}{\mu} \begin{pmatrix} \frac{\nu(x+1)}{d_{x+1}} & 0 \\ 0 & \frac{\nu(x+1)}{c_{x+1}} \end{pmatrix} \begin{pmatrix} \frac{\kappa(x)+\mu}{c_x} & 1 \\ \frac{\kappa(x)}{c_x} & 1 \end{pmatrix} \\
&= \frac{c_x}{\mu} \begin{pmatrix} \frac{(\kappa(x)+\mu)\nu(x+1)}{c_x d_{x+1}} & \frac{\nu(x+1)}{d_{x+1}} \\ \frac{\kappa(x)\nu(x+1)}{c_x c_{x+1}} & \frac{\nu(x+1)}{c_{x+1}} \end{pmatrix},
\end{aligned}
$$

as required.

The steady state distribution

Set $w_M := (\kappa(M)/c_M, 1)$. Let $\tilde{\pi}_x = (\tilde{\pi}_x(0), \tilde{\pi}_x(1))$ be defined as

$$
\tilde{\pi}_x = w_M \alpha_{M-1} \alpha_{M-2} \cdots \alpha_x / \tilde{Z}_M,
$$

$$
\tilde{\pi}_M = w_M / \tilde{Z}_M,
$$

where $\tilde{Z}_M$ is the normalisation constant

$$
\tilde{Z}_M = w_M \Big(\sum_{j=0}^{M-1} \alpha_{M-1} \cdots \alpha_j \Big) \mathbf{1} + w_M \mathbf{1}, \text{ and } \mathbf{1} = (1,1)'.
$$

When $\mu_0 = 0$, the steady state $\pi_x = (\pi_x(0), \pi_x(1))$ is

$$
\pi_x = \Big(\frac{\tilde{\pi}_x(0)}{d_x Z_M}, \frac{\tilde{\pi}_x(1)}{c_x Z_M} \Big),
$$

where Z_M is the normalization constant

$$
Z_M = \sum_{x=0}^{M} \Big(\frac{\tilde{\pi}_x(0)}{d_x} + \frac{\tilde{\pi}_x(1)}{c_x} \Big).
$$

A.3.1 Stochastic simulations with MATLAB®

The following Matlab commands provide a way of simulating the self-regulated gene.

```
function [N,Y]=simul_selfreg(mu,alpha,nu,beta,g,g0,kappa,S,T)
```

```
%%%%%%%%%%%%%%%%%%%%%%%%%%%%%%%%%%%%%%%%%%%%%%%%%%%%%
% Simulation for the self-regulated gene network

%  N = protein number
%  Switch ON/OFF rate: kappa
%  Switch OFF/ON rate : g*N^5 + g0
%  Production rate  in ON state : mu
%  Production rate in OFF state for N>0: alpha*mu
%  Production rate in OFF state for N=0: mu
%  Degradation rate : nu*(N-beta*N/2)
%%%%%%%%%%%%%%%%%%%%%%%%%%%%%%%%%%%%%%%%%%%%%%%%%%%%%


%%%%%%%%%%%%%%%%%%%%%%%%%%%%%%%%%%%%%%%%%%%%%%%%%%%%%
% Parameters:
%
% mu          protein production rate(promoter ON)
% alpha       proportion coefficient
% nu          protein degradation parameter
% beta      parameter for degradation
% g       OFF/ON switch
% g0       basal OFF/ON switch
% kappa      ON/OFF switch

% S           number of simulations
% T           number of trajectories



% initialisation
% N           number of proteins
% Y           promoter state : 0-> OFF, 1-> ON

N=round(10*rand(T,1));
Y=round(rand(T,1));

S0=floor(9*S/10);
k=1;
```

```
while k<S0+1


  taux=[kappa.*Y,g.*(1-Y).*N.^5+g0*(1-Y),mu.*Y

  +alpha*mu.*(1-Y)+mu.*(1-Y).*(N==0),nu.*(N-beta*N./2)];
  somme=cumsum(taux,2);
  U=rand (T,1).*sum(taux,2);
  Y=Y-indicatrice(zeros(T,1),somme(:,1),U)

  +indicatrice(somme(:,1),somme(:,2),U);
  N=N+indicatrice(somme(:,2),somme(:,3),U)

  -indicatrice(somme(:,3),somme(:,4),U);
  k=k+1;
end

% we save only the last 10% of the simulation
k=1;

while k<S-S0+1

  taux=[kappa.*Y(:,k),g.*(1-Y(:,k)).*N (:,k).^5

  +g0*(1-Y(:,k)),mu.*Y(:,k)

  +alpha*mu.*(1-Y(:,k))+mu.*(1-Y(:,k)).*(N(:,k)==0),nu.*(N(:,k)

  -beta*N (:,k)./2)];
  somme=cumsum(taux,2);
  U=rand (T,1).*sum(taux,2);
  Y(:,k+1)=Y(:,k)-indicatrice(zeros(T,1),somme(:,1),U)

  +indicatrice(somme(:,1),somme(:,2),U);
  N(:,k+1)=N(:,k)+indicatrice(somme(:,2),somme(:,3),U)

  -indicatrice(somme(:,3),somme(:,4),U);
```

```
    k=k+1;


end
```

The following list of MATLAB commands lead to the computation of the stationary distribution associated with the self-regulated gene:

```
% Parameters
mu=650;
nu=150;
g=0.5;
g0=150;
kappa=200;
alpha=0.1;
beta=0.4;

[N,Y]=simul_selfreg(mu,alpha,nu,beta,g,g0,kappa,30000,10);

freq=mc_strip(N,Y);


% Computing the invariant measure of the
% time-continuous Markov chain

n=length(freq);

Qi=zeros(n,2);
Qi(:,1)=g.*(0:(n-1))'.^5+g0+alpha*mu +nu.*((0:(n-1))'-beta*(0:(n-1))'));
Qi(:,2)=kappa+mu+nu.*((0:(n-1))'-beta*(0:(n-1))'));
Qi(1,1)=Qi(1,1)+mu;
```

```
pitilde=freq./Qi;
beta=1/sum(sum(pitilde));
pi=beta*pitilde;


figure()
I=(0:(length(pi)-1))';
b1=bar(I,pi(:,1),0.5,'facecolor',[.7,.7,.7]);
hold on
b2=bar(I+0.5,pi(:,2),0.5,'facecolor','k');
xlabel('Number of proteins','FontSize',12)
ylabel('Probability','FontSize',12)
axis([-0.5 length(pi) 0 0.14])
```

The following functions are used in the above MATLAB codes. The first one allows the computation of indicator functions, and the second one furnishes empirical frequencies associated with the Markov chain modelling the self-regulated gene:

```
function c=indicatrice(a,b,x)

% a,b : interval limits
% x : test variable

if prod(x-a)*prod(x-b)==0
    c=zeros(size(x));
    for k=1:length(x)
        if x(k)>=a(k) & x(k)<b(k)
            c(k)=1;
        end
    end
else
    c=heaviside (x-a).*(1-heaviside(x-b));
end



function frq=mc_strip(x,y) % x : vector or matrix
```

```
% x -> matrix containing the number of proteins in the ON/OFF  states
% y -> matrix associated with the promoter's state

frq=zeros(max(max(x)),2);
for k=0:max(max(x))
    frq(k+1,1)=sum(sum(x(y==0)==k)); % empirical frequency
    frq(k+1,2)=sum(sum(x(y==1)==k));
end
N=numel(x);
frq=frq/N;
```

Appendix B

Asymptotic behaviour of the solutions to time-continuous Lyapunov equations

B.1 Time-continuous Lyapunov equations

Section 12.1 introduces density dependent processes where a law of large numbers leads to the o.d.e.

$$\frac{\mathrm{d}\bar{X}(s)}{\mathrm{d}s} = F(\bar{X}(s)), \tag{B.1}$$

$\bar{X}(0) = x_0$. Section 12.4 focuses on the same setting by producing gaussian approximations, where the covariance function $\Sigma(t)$ solves the time-continuous Lyapunov equation (12.12)

$$\frac{\mathrm{d}\Sigma(t)}{\mathrm{d}t} = \mathrm{D}F(\bar{X}(t))\Sigma(t) + \Sigma(t)\mathrm{D}F(\bar{X}(t))^T + G(\bar{X}(t)). \tag{B.2}$$

The aim of this section is to give some properties of such equations when the orbit of the above o.d.e. starts in the vicinity of an asymptotically stable equilibrium $\bar{X}_*$ of (B.1). We hence assume that the matrices

$$K(t) = \mathrm{D}F(\bar{X}(t))$$

are stable, with

$$\sup_{\lambda \in \mathrm{Spec}(K(t))} \Re(\lambda) < 0. \tag{B.3}$$

When $\bar{X}(t) \to \bar{X}_*$ as $t \to \infty$,

$$K(t) \longrightarrow K = \mathrm{D}F(\bar{X}_*) \text{ and } G(\bar{X}(t)) \longrightarrow G.$$

Our aim is to give sufficient conditions on these matrices ensuring that $\Sigma(t)$ converges toward a limiting covariance matrix Σ which solves the Lyapunov equation

$$KΣ + ΣK^T + G = 0,$$

which has a unique positive-definite solution $Σ$ when G is positive definite and K is stable; see, e.g., [63] or [105], or theorem B.2.3.

Recall that the tensor product $B ⊗ C$ is

$$B ⊗ C = \begin{pmatrix} b_{11}C & b_{12}C & \cdots & b_{1n}C \\ b_{21}C & b_{22}C & \cdots & b_{2n}C \\ \cdots & \cdots & \cdots & \cdots \\ b_{n1}C & b_{n2}C & \cdots & b_{nn}C \end{pmatrix}.$$

Moreover, let $B(i)$ denote the ith column of B; then

$$\text{col}(B) = \begin{pmatrix} B(1) \\ B(2) \\ \cdots \\ B(n) \end{pmatrix}.$$

One can recast (B.2) as a nonhomogeneous linear differential equation

$$\frac{dA(t)}{dt} = \mathcal{K}(t)A(t) + H(t), \tag{B.4}$$

where $\mathcal{K}(t) = K(t) ⊗ \text{id} + \text{id} ⊗ K(t)$, $A(t) = \text{col}(Σ(t))$ and $H(t) = \text{col}(G(\bar{X}(t)))$. Notice that the spectrum of $\mathcal{K}(t)$ is composed of the sums $λ_i(t) + λ_j(t)$, where the $λ_i(t)$ and $λ_j(t)$ denote the eigenvalues of $K(t)$; see, e.g., [62].

B.2   Asymptotically autonomous dynamical systems

The differential equation (B.4) is asymptotically constant since both $\mathcal{K}(t)$ and $H(t)$ converge toward limiting constant matrices $\mathcal{K}(∞)$ and $H(∞)$, when the trajectory $\bar{X}(t)$ starts in the neighbourhood of an asymptotically stable equilibrium $\bar{X}_*$. We introduce some notions from dynamical system theory which will be useful to get results on such asymptotically autonomous dynamical systems. We follow essentially [14]. Section 9.5 introduces the notion of flow; in our setting, we use the notion of semiflow $Φ$, which is similarly defined by a continuous map on a metric space (M, d) such that

$$Φ : M × \mathbb{R}_+ → M,$$

$$(x, t) \mapsto \Phi_t(x).$$

(i) $\Phi_0 = \mathrm{Id}$.

(ii) For all $t, s \in \mathbb{R}_+$

$$\Phi_t \circ \Phi_s = \Phi_{t+s}.$$

A continuous function $X : \mathbb{R}_+ \to M$ is an **asymptotic pseudotrajectory** for Φ if

$$\lim_{t \to \infty} d(X(t + T), \Phi_T(X(t))) = 0,$$

locally uniformly in $T \in \mathbb{R}_+$. In this case, for each fixed $s > 0$, the curve

$$[0, s] \to M, \ t \mapsto X(t + T)$$

shadows the Φ-trajectory of the point $X(T)$ over the interval $[0, s]$ with arbitrary accuracy when T is large. X is said to be **precompact** if its image has compact closure in M. The **limit set** $L\{X\}$ of an asymptotic pseudotrajectory X is

$$L\{X\} = \cap_{t \geq 0} \overline{X[t, \infty]}.$$

The following results can be found in [14]: If $K \subset M$ is an invariant set for Φ, we say that K is *internally chain recurrent* if the restriction $\Phi|_K$ is chain recurrent, that is, if $\Phi|_K$ has no proper attractor.

Theorem B.2.1 $L\{X\}$ *is Φ-invariant, connected, compact and internally chain recurrent*

Let $g : \mathbb{R}^n \to \mathbb{R}^n$ and $f : \mathbb{R}_+ \times \mathbb{R}^n \to \mathbb{R}^n$ be continuous maps. The o.d.e.

$$\frac{\mathrm{d}x}{\mathrm{d}t} = f(t, x) \tag{B.5}$$

is called **asymptotically autonomous** with limit equation

$$\frac{\mathrm{d}x}{\mathrm{d}t} = g(x), \tag{B.6}$$

if

$$\lim_{t \to \infty} f(t, x) = g(x),$$

locally uniformly in x.

Theorem B.2.2 *Let X be a bounded solution to (B.5), and let Φ be the flow generated by (B.6). Then X is an asymptotic pseudotrajectory of Φ.*

We will need the following theorem; see, e.g., [110], section 17, or [105], section 4.3:

Theorem B.2.3 *Consider the Lyapunov equation*

$$KP + PK^T + Q = 0, \tag{B.7}$$

where Q is a symmetric matrix. Then K is stable, that is, $\Re(\lambda) < 0$, $\forall \lambda \in$ Spec(K), if and only if given any positive definite matrix Q there exists a positive definite symmetric matrix P that satisfies (B.7). Moreover, if K is stable, then P is the unique solution of (B.7).

The following result gives the asymptotic behaviour of the solutions to (B.2):

Theorem B.2.4 *Let $\bar{X}(t)$ be a solution of the o.d.e. (B.1), which starts in the basin of attraction of an asymptotically stable equilibrium point $\bar{X}_*$. Then, the solution $\Sigma(t)$ of (B.2) is an asymptotic pseudotrajectory of the flow associated with the autonomous o.d.e.*

$$\frac{d\Sigma(t)}{dt} = K\Sigma(t) + \Sigma(t)K^T + G, \tag{B.8}$$

where the constant matrices K and G are such that

$$K = \lim_{t \to \infty} K(\bar{X}(t)) \text{ and } G = \lim_{t \to \infty} G(\bar{X}(t)).$$

Suppose moreover that G is symmetric and positive definite, and that

$$\sup_{t \geq 0} \sup_{\lambda \in \text{Spec}(K(t))} \Re(\lambda) < -a < 0, \tag{B.9}$$

for some positive constant $a > 0$. Then, the solution $\Sigma(t)$ of (B.2) converges toward the unique covariance matrix Σ which solves the Lyapunov equation

$$K\Sigma + \Sigma K^T + G = 0.$$

PROOF:

Let A be a solution of B.2. For a matrix B, let $B^H = (A + A^T)/2$ be the Hermitian part of B, and let $\beta^0(t)$ be the largest (real) eigenvalue of $\mathcal{K}^H(t)$. Classical results on o.d.e. show that

$$||A(t)|| \leq ||A(0)|| \exp\left(\int_0^t \beta^0(s)ds\right)$$
$$+ \int_0^t ||H(s)|| \exp\left(\int_s^t \beta^0(r)dr\right)ds;$$

see, e.g., [78], Lemma 4.20. This implies that $A(t)$ is bounded: from construction, $H(s) = \mathrm{col}(G(\bar{X}(s)))$, and $\bar{X}(s)$ starts in the neighbourhood of an asymptotically stable equilibrium, with $\bar{X}(t) \to \bar{X}_*$ as $t \to \infty$. Moreover, by assumption

$$\beta^0(r) \leq -a < 0, \ \forall r.$$

Theorem B.2.2 shows that $A(t)$ is an asymptotic pseudotrajectory of the autonomous o.d.e.

$$\frac{\mathrm{d}B(t)}{\mathrm{d}t} = \mathcal{K}(\infty)B(t) + H(\infty), \tag{B.10}$$

where

$$\mathcal{K}(\infty) = K \otimes \mathrm{id} + \mathrm{id} \otimes K.$$

The eigenvalues of $\mathcal{K}(\infty)$ are the sums $\lambda_i(\infty) + \lambda_j(\infty)$ of the eigenvalues of K, whose real parts are bounded by $-a < 0$ from hypothesis. The equilibria $B(\infty) = \mathrm{col}(\Sigma(\infty))$ of the linear o.d.e. (B.10) satisfy

$$\mathcal{K}(\infty)B + H(\infty) = 0,$$

or equivalently

$$K\Sigma(\infty) + \Sigma(\infty)K^T + G = 0,$$

which possess a unique symmetric and positive definite solution $\Sigma(\infty)$ when G is symmetric and positive definite; see theorem B.2.3. Theorem B.2.1 states that the limit set $L\{A\}$ of the asymptotic pseudotrajectory A is Φ-invariant, where Φ is the flow associated with (B.10), and we hence deduce that

$$L\{A\} = \{\Sigma(\infty)\},$$

as required. $\square$

.

Bibliography

[1] E. Aarts and J. Korst. *Simulated Annealing and Boltzmann Machines.* Wiley, 1989.

[2] G. Ackers, D. Johnson, and M. Shea. Quantitative model for gene regulation by λ phage repressor. *PNAS*, 79:1129–1133, 1982.

[3] L. Allen. *An Introduction to Stochastic Processes with Applications to Biology.* Chapman and Hall CRC, 2011.

[4] U. Alon. *An Introduction to Systems Biology: Design Principles of Biological Circuits.* Chapman & Hall/CRC, 2007.

[5] D. Anderson, G. Craciun, and T. Kurtz. Product-form stationary distributions for deficiency zero chemical reaction networks. *Bul. Math. Biol.*, 72:1947–1970, 2010.

[6] D. Anderson and T. Kurtz. Continuous Time Markov Chain Models for Chemical Reaction Networks. In Design and Analysis of Biomolecular Circuits, H. Koeppl, D. Densmore, G. Setti, M. di Bernardo, eds., pages 3–42, 2011.

[7] A. Arkin, J. Ross, and H. McAdams. Stochastic kinetic analysis of developmental pathway bifurcation in phage λ-infected *Escherichia coli* cells. *Genetics*, 149:1633–1648, 1998.

[8] D. Austin, M. Allen, J. McCollum, J. Wilgus, G. Sayler, N. Samatova, C. Cox, and M. Simpson. Gene networks shaping of inherent noise spectra. *Nature*, 439:608–611, 2006.

[9] N. Bailey. *The Elements of Stochastic Processes.* Wiley, 1964.

[10] D. Beard and H. Qian. *Chemical Biophysics: Quantitative Analysis of Cellular Systems.* Cambridge. Cambridge University Press, 2008.

[11] A. Becskei, B. Seraphin, and L. Serrano. Positive feedback in eukaryotic gene networks: cell differentiation by graded to binary response conversion. *EMBO J.*, 20:2528–2535, 2001.

[12] A. Becskei and L. Serrano. Engineering stability in gene networks by autoregulation. *Nature*, 405:590–593, 2000.

[13] M. Behar, N. Hao, H. Dohlman, and T. Elston. Mathematical and computational analysis of adaptation via feedback inhibition in signal transduction pathways. *Biophy. J.*, 93:806–821, 2007.

[14] M. Benaïm and M. Hirsch. Asymptotic pseudotrajectories and chain recurrent flows, with applications. *J. Dynamics. Diff. Equ.*, 8:141–176, 1996.

[15] P. Benos, M. Bulyk, and G. Stormo. Additivity in protein-DNA interactions: how good an approximation is it? *Nucl. Acid. Res.*, 30:4442–4451, 2002.

[16] O. Berg. A model for the statistical fluctuations of protein numbers in a microbial population. *J. Theor. Biol.*, 71:587–603, 1978.

[17] O. Berg and P. von Hippel. Selection of DNA binding sites by regulatory proteins. Statistical-mechanical theory and applications to operators and promoters. *J. Mol. Biol.*, 193:723–750, 1987.

[18] N. Biggs. Algebraic potential theory on graphs. *Bul. London Math. Soc.*, 29:641–682, 1997.

[19] L. Bintu, N. Buchler, H. Garcia, U. Gerland, T. Hwa, J. Kondev, T. Kuhlman, and R. Phillips. Transcriptional regulation by the numbers: applications. *Curr. Op. Gen. Dev.*, 15:125–135, 2005.

[20] L. Bintu, N. Buchler, H. Garcia, U. Gerland, T. Hwa, J. Kondev, T. Kuhlman, and R. Phillips. Transcriptional regulation by the numbers: models. *Curr. Op. Gen. Dev.*, 15:116–124, 2005.

[21] H. Black. Stabilized feedback amplifiers. *Bell Syst. Tech. J.*, 13:1–18, 1934.

[22] W. Blake, G. Balazsi, M.A. Kohanski, F.J. Issacs, K.F. Murphy, Y. Kuang, C.R. Cantor, D.R. Walt, and J. Collins. Gene expression. *Mol. Cell*, 24:853–865, 2006.

[23] E. Bolthausen and I. Goldscheid. Recurrence and transience of random walks in random environments. *Commun. Math. Phys.*, 214:429–447, 2000.

[24] R. Bott and J.P. Mayberry. *Matrices and Trees. Economic Activity Analysis.* Wiley, New York, 1954.

[25] C. Bowsher, M. Voliotis, and P. Swain. The fidelity of dynamic signaling by noisy biomolecular networks. *Plos Comput. Biol.*, 9:e1002965, 2013.

[26] P. Bucher. Weight matrix description of four eukaryotic RNA polymerase II promoter elements derived from 502 unrelated promoters. *J. Mol. Biol.*, 212:563–578, 1990.

[27] N. Buchler, U. Gerland, and T. Hwa. On schemes of combinatorial transcription logic. *PNAS*, 100:5136–5141, 2003.

[28] Y. Cao, D. Gillespie, and L. Petzold. The slow scale stochastic simulation algorithm. *J. Chem. Phys.*, 122:014116, 2005.

[29] M. Chaves, E. Sontag, and R. Dinerstein. Optimal length and signal amplification in weakly activated signal transduction cascades. *J. Phys. Chem.*, 108:15311–15320, 2004.

[30] O. Ciquin and J. Domongeot. Roles of positive and negative feedback in biological systems. *C.R. Biologies*, 325:1085–1095, 2002.

[31] B. Clarke. Stability of complex reaction networks. *Adv. Chem. Phys.*, 43:1–217, 1975.

[32] C. Conradi and D. Flockerzi. Multistationarity in mass action networks with applications to ERK activation. *J. Math. Biol.*, 65:107–156, 2012.

[33] G. Craciun and M. Feinberg. Multiple equilibria in complex chemical reaction networks: I. The injectivity property. *SIAM J. Appl. Math.*, 5:1526–1546, 2005.

[34] G. Craciun and M. Feinberg. Multiple equilibria in complex chemical reaction networks: II. The species-reaction graph. *SIAM J. Appl. Math.*, 4:1321–1338, 2006.

[35] G. Craciun and M. Feinberg. Multiple equilibria in complex chemical reaction networks: semiopen mass action systems. *SIAM J. Appl. Math.*, 70:1859–1877, 2010.

[36] I. Darvey, B.W. Ninham, and P.J. Staff. Stochastic models for second-order chemical reaction kinetics. The equilibrium state. *J. Chem. Phys.*, 45:2145, 1966.

[37] I.G. Darvey and P.J. Staff. Stochastic approach to first-order chemical reactions kinetics. *J.Chem.Phys.*, 44:990, 1966.

[38] M. Delbrück. Statistical fluctuations in autocatalytic reactions. *J. Chem. Phys.*, 8:120–124, 1940.

[39] A. Dembo and O. Zeitouni. *Large Deviations Techniques and Applications.* Springer, New York, 2009.

[40] E. Di Cera. *Thermodynamic Theory of Site-Specific Binding Processes in Biological Macromolecules.* Cambridge University Press, 1995.

[41] K. Dill and S. Bromberg. *Molecular Driving Forces.* Garland Science, 2003.

[42] M. Domijan and E. Pécou. The interaction graph structure of mass-action reaction networks. *J. Math. Biol.*, 65:375–402, 2012.

[43] J. Elf and M. Ehrenberg. Fast evaluation of fluctuations in biochemical networks with the linear noise approximation. *Genome Res.*, 13:2475–2484, 2003.

[44] J. Elf, J. Paulsson, O. Berg, and M. Ehrenberg. Near-critical phenomena in intracellular metabolite pools. *Biophy. J.*, 84:154–170, 2003.

[45] R. Ellis. *Entropy, Large Deviations and Statistical Mechanics*. Springer, New York, 1985.

[46] M. Elowitz, A. Levine, E. Siggia, and P. Swain. Stochastic gene expression in a single cell. *Science*, 297:1183–1186, 2002.

[47] S. Ethier and T. Kurtz. *Markov Processes: Characterization and Convergence*. Wiley, New York, 1986.

[48] M. Feinberg. Complex balancing in general kinetic systems. *Arch. Rat. Mech. Anal.*, 49:187–194, 1972.

[49] M. Feinberg. Lectures on Chemical Reaction Networks. *Lecture Notes, Mathematics Research Center, University of Wisconsin-Madison*, 1979.

[50] M. Feinberg. Necessary and sufficient conditions for detailed balancing in mass action systems of arbitrary complexity. *Chem. Eng. Sci.*, 44:1819–1827, 1989.

[51] M. Feinberg. Existence and uniqueness of steady states for a class of chemical reaction networks. *Arch. Rat. Mech. Anal.*, 132:311–370, 1995.

[52] J. Ferrell. Self-perpetuating states in signal transductions: positive feedback, double-negative feedback and bistability. *Curr. Opinion in Chem. Biol.*, 6:140–148, 2002.

[53] J. Ferrell, J. Pomerening, S. Kim, N. Trunnell, W. Xiong, C. Huang, and E. Machleder. Simple, realistic models of complex biological processes: Positive feedback and bistability in a cell fate switch and a cell cycle oscillator. *FEBS Lett.*, 583:3999–4005, 2009.

[54] B. Flury. *A First Course in Multivariate Analysis*. Springer, New York, 1997.

[55] D. Forger and C. Peskin. Stochastic simulation of the mammalian circadian clock. *PNAS*, 102:321–324, 2005.

[56] C. Fortuin, P. Kasteleyn, and J. Ginibre. Correlation inequalities on some partially ordered sets. *Comm. Math. Phys.*, 22:80–103, 1971.

[57] T. Fournier, J.P. Gabriel, C. Mazza, J. Pasquier, J.L. Galbete, and N. Mermod. Steady state expression of self-regulated genes. *Bioinformatics*, 23:3185–3192, 2007.

[58] T. Fournier, J.P. Gabriel, C. Mazza, J. Pasquier, J.L. Galbete, and N. Mermod. Stochastic models and numerical algorithms for a class of regulatory gene networks. *Bull. Math. Bio.*, 71:1394–1431, 2009.

[59] D. Freedman. *Markov Chains*. Holden Day, San Francisco, 1971.

[60] M.I. Freidlin and A.D. Wentzell. *Random Perturbations of Dynamical Systems*. Springer, Berlin, 1984.

[61] A. Frost. Effect of concentration on reaction rate and equilibrium. *J. Chem. Educ.*, 18:272, 1941.

[62] C. Gadgil, C. Lee, and H. Othmer. A stochastic analysis of first-order reaction networks. *Bull. Math. Bio.*, 67:901–946, 2005.

[63] Z. Gajic, M. Tahir, and J. Qureshi. *Lyapunov Matrix Equation in System Stability and Control*. Academic Press, San Diego, 1995.

[64] D. Gale and H. Nikaido. The Jacobian matrix and global univalence of mappings. *Math. Ann.*, 159:81–93, 1965.

[65] D. Gillespie. A general method for numerically simulating the stochastic time evolution of coupled chemical reactions. *J. Comp. Phys.*, 22:403–434, 1976.

[66] D. Gillespie. Exact stochastic simulation of coupled chemical reactions. *J. Chem. Phys.*, 81:2340–2361, 1977.

[67] D. Gillespie. Approximate accelerated stochastic simulation of chemically reacting systems. *J. Chem. Phys.*, 122:1716–1733, 2001.

[68] M. E. Gilpin. Spiral chaos in a predator-prey model. *Amer. Nat.*, 113:306–308, 179.

[69] S. Glasstone, K. Ladler, and H. Eyring. *The Theory of Rate Processes: The Kinetics of Chemical Reactions, Viscosity, Diffusion and Electrochemical Phenomena*. McGraw-Hill, New-York, 1941.

[70] A. Goldbetter and D. Koshland. An amplified sensitivity arising from covalent modifications in biological systems. *PNAS*, 78:6840–6844, 1981.

[71] J.L. Gouze. Positive and negative circuits in dynamical systems. *J. Biol. Syst.*, 6:11–15, 1998.

[72] C. Govern and A. Chakraborty. Signaling cascades modulate the speed of signal propagation through space. *Plos One*, 4:4639, 2009.

[73] S. Grossinsky, G. Schütz, and H. Spohn. Condensation in the zero range process: stationary and dynamical properties. *J. Stat. Phys.*, 113:389–410, 2003.

[74] N. Guido, X. Wang, D. Adalsteinsson, D. McMillen, J. Hasty, C. Cantor, T. Elston, and J. Collins. A bottom-up approach to gene regulation. *Nature*, 439:856–860, 2006.

[75] J. Gunawardena. Chemical reaction networks theory for in-silico biologists. *Lecture Notes, Bauer Center for Genomic Research, Harvard University*, 2003.

[76] J. Gunawardena. Multisite protein phosphorylation makes a good threshold but can be a poor switch. *PNAS*, 102:14617–14622, 2005.

[77] T. Harris. A lower bound for the critical probability in a certain percolation process. *Proc. Cambridge Phil. Soc.*, 56:13–20, 1960.

[78] P. Hartman. *Ordinary Differential Equations*. Classics In Applied Mathematics. SIAM, 2002.

[79] P. Hartmann. *Ordinary Differential Equations*. Wiley, New York, 1964.

[80] W. Hastings. Monte Carlo sampling methods using Markov chains and their applications. *Biometrika*, 57:97–109, 1970.

[81] J. Hasty, J. Pradines, M. Dolnik, and J. Collins. Noise-based switches and amplifiers for gene expression. *PNAS*, 97:2075–2080, 2000.

[82] V. Hatzimanikatis, C. Li, J. Ionita, C. Henry, M. Jankowski, and L. Broadbelt. Exploring the diversity of complex metabolic networks. *Bioinformatics*, 21:1603–1609, 2004.

[83] R. Heinrich, G. Neel, and T. Rapoport. Mathematical models of protein kinase signal transduction. *Mol. Cell*, 9:957–970, 2002.

[84] A. Hill. The possible effect of the aggregation of the molecules of haemoglobin on its dissociation curves. *J. Physiol. London*, 40:Suppl. iv–vii, 1910.

[85] M. W. Hirsch and S. Smale. *Differential Equations, Dynamical Systems, and Linear Algebra*, volume 60 of *Pure and Applied Mathematics*. Academic Press, 1974.

[86] M. W. Hirsch, S. Smale, and R. L. Devaney. *Differential Equations, Dynamical Systems and An Introduction to Chaos*. Elsevier Academic Press, Amsterdam, 2004.

[87] J. Hofbauer and K. Sigmung. *Evolutionary Games and Population Dynamics*. Cambridge University Press, Cambridge, 1998.

[88] K. Holstein, D. Flockerzi, and C. Conradi. Multistationarity in sequential distributed multisite phosphorylation networks. *Bull. Math. Biol.*, 75:2028–2058, 2013.

[89] F. Horn. Necessary and sufficient conditions for complex balancing in chemical kinetics. *Arch. Rat. Mech. Anal.*, 49:172–186, 1972.

[90] F. Horn and R. Jackson. General mass action kinetics. *Arch. Rat. Mech. Anal.*, 47:81–116, 1972.

[91] S. Huang. The molecular and mathematical basis of Waddington's epigenetic landscape: A framework for post-Darwinian biology? *Bioessays*, 34:149–157, 2011.

[92] F. Isaacs, J. Hasty, C. Cantor, and J. Collins. Prediction and measurment of an autoregulatory genetic module. *PNAS*, 100:7714–7719, 2003.

[93] A. Ivanova. Conditions for the uniqueness of the stationary states of kinetic systems, connected with the structures of their reaction mechanisms. *Kinet. Katal.*, 20:1019–1023, 1979.

[94] A. Ivanova. One approach to the determination of a number of qualitative features in the behaviour of kinetic systems, and realization of this approach in a computer (critical conditions, autooscillations). *Kinet. Katal.*, 20:1541–1548, 1979.

[95] F. Jacob and J. Monod. Genetic regulatory mechanisms in the synthesis of proteins. *J. Mol. Biol.*, 3:318–356, 1961.

[96] S. Karlin. Measures of enzyme's cooperativity. *J. Theoret. Biol.*, 85:33–54, 1980.

[97] S. Karlin and R. Kenett. Shapes of velocity curves in multiunit enzyme kinetic systems. *Math. Biosci.*, 52:97–115, 1980.

[98] J. Karr, J. Sanghvi, D. Macklin, V. Gutschow, J. Jacobs, B. Bolival, N. Assad-Garcia, J. Glass, and M. Covert. A whole-cell computational model predicts phenotype from genotype. *Cell*, 150:389–401, 2012.

[99] M. Kaufman, C. Soulé, and R. Thomas. A new necessary condition on interaction graphs for multistationarity. *J. Theor. Biol.*, 248:675–685, 2007.

[100] M. Kaufman and R. Thomas. Model analysis of the bases of multistationarity in the humoral immune response. *J. Theor. Biol.*, 129:141–162, 1987.

[101] A. Keller. Model genetic circuits encoding autoregulatory transcription factors. *J. Theor. Biol.*, 172:169–185, 1995.

[102] F. Kelly. *Reversibility and Stochastic Networks*. Wiley, New York, 1979.

[103] D. Kennell and H. Riezman. Transcription and translation initiation frequencies of the *Escherichia coli* lac operon. *J. Mol. Biol.*, 114:1–21, 1977.

[104] T. Kepler and T. Elston. Stochasticity in transcriptional regulation: Origins, consequences and mathematical representations. *Bioph. J.*, 81:3116–3136, 2001.

[105] H. Khalil. *Nonlinear Systems*. Prentice Hall, Upper Saddle River, 2000.

[106] B. Kholodenko. Cell-signalling dynamics in time and space. *Nat. Rev. Mol. Cell Biol.*, 7:165–176, 2006.

[107] C. Kipnis and C. Landim. *Scaling Limits of Interacting Particle Systems*. Springer, Berlin, 1995.

[108] P. Kirk, T. Toni, and M. Stumpf. Parameter inference for biochemical systems that undergo a Hopf bifurcation. *Bioph. J.*, 95:540–549, 2008.

[109] D. Koshland, G. Nemethy, and D. Filmer. Comparison of experimental binding data and theoretical models in proteins containing subunits. *Biochem.*, 5:365, 1966.

[110] J. La Salle and S. Lefschetz. *Stability by Liapunov's Direct Method*. Academic Press, Baltimore, 1961.

[111] J. Lebowitz. GHS and other inequalities. *Commun. Math. Phys.*, 35:87–92, 1974.

[112] C. Lee and H. Othmer. A multi-scale analysis of chemical reaction networks: I. Deterministic systems. *J. Math. Biol.*, 60:387–450, 2010.

[113] I. Lestas, G. Vinnicombe, and J. Paulsson. Fundamental limits on the suppression of molecular fluctuations. *Nature*, 467:174–178, 2010.

[114] E. Levine and T. Hwa. Stochastic fluctuations in metabolic pathways. *PNAS*, 104:9224–9229, 2007.

[115] X. Liu, L. Bardwell, and Q. Nie. A combination of multisite phosphorylation and substrate sequestration produces switchinglike responses. *Bioph. J.*, 98:1396–1407, 2010.

[116] W. Ma, A. Trusina, H. El-Samad, W. Lim, and C. Tang. Defining network topologies that can achieve biochemical adaptation. *Cell*, 138:760–773, 2009.

[117] C. Maeder, M. Hink, A. Kinkhabwala, P. Mayr, H. Bastiaens, and M. Korp. Spatial regulation of Fus3 MAP kinase activity through a reaction-diffusion mechanism in yeast pheromone signalling. *Nature Cell Biology*, 9:1319–1326, 2007.

[118] G. Manning, D. Whyte, R. Martinez, T. Hunter, and S. Sudarsanam. The protein kinase complement of the human genome. *Science*, 298:1912–1934, 2002.

[119] N. Markevich, J. Hoek, and B. Kholodenko. Signaling switches and bistability arising from multisite phosphorylation in protein kianse cascades. *J. Cell. Biol.*, 164:353–359, 2004.

[120] F. Marks, U. Müller, and K. Müller-Decker. *Cellular Signal Processing. An Introduction to the Molecular Mechanisms of Signal Transduction.* Garland Science, Taylor and Francis Group, 2009.

[121] B. Martins and P. Swain. Ultrasensitivity in phosphorylation-dephosphorylation cycles with litle substrate. *Plos Comput. Biol.*, 9:e1003175, 2013.

[122] R. M. May and W. Leonard. Nonlinear aspects of competition between three species. *Siam J. Appl. Math*, 29:243–252, 1975.

[123] J. Maybee and J. Quirk. Qualitative problems in matrix theory. *SIAM Rev.*, 11:30–51, 1969.

[124] H. McAdams and A. Arkin. Stochastic mechanisms in gene expression. *PNAS*, 94:814–819, 1997.

[125] D. McQuarrie. Stochastic approach to chemical kinetics. *J. Appl. Probab.*, 85:413–478, 1967.

[126] N. Metropolis, A. Rosenbluth, M. Rosenbluth, A. Teller, and E. Teller. Equations of state calculations by fast computing machines. *J. Chem. Phys.*, 21:1087–1091, 1953.

[127] G Michal. *Biochemical Pathways*. Spektrum, Akad. Verl., Heidelberg, 1999.

[128] M. Mincheva and G. Craciun. Multigraph conditions for multistability, oscillations and pattern formation in biochemical reaction networks. *Proc. IEEE*, 96:1281–1291, 2008.

[129] M. Mincheva and M. Rossel. Graph-theoretic methods for the analysis of chemical and biochemical networks. I. Multistability and oscillations in ordinary differential equations models. *J. Math. Biol.*, 55:61–86, 2007.

[130] L. Mirny. Nucleosome-mediated cooperativity between transcription factors. *PNAS*, 107:22534–22539, 2010.

[131] J. Monod, J. Wyman, and J. Changeux. On the nature of the allosteric transitions: A plausible model. *J. Molec. Biol.*, 12:88–118, 1965.

[132] B. Müller-Hill. *The lac Operon: A Short History of a Genetic Paradigm.* Walter De Gruyter, Berlin, 1996.

[133] J. R. Norris. *Markov Chains*. Cambridge University Press, Cambridge., 1997.

[134] E. Ozbudak, M. Thattai, I. Kurtser, A. Grossman, and A. van Oude-naarden. Regulation of noise in the expression of a single gene. *Nature Genet.*, 31:69–73, 2005.

[135] B. Palsson. *Systems Biology. Properties of Reconstructed Networks*. Cambridge University Press, Cambridge, 2006.

[136] G. Palumbo and S. Pennisi. *Feedback Amplifiers: Theory and Design*. Kluwer Academic, Boston/Dordrecht/London, 2002.

[137] J. Paulsson. Summing up the noise in gene networks. *Nature*, 427:415–418, 2004.

[138] J. Paulsson. Models of stochastic gene expression. *Phys. Life Rev.*, 2:157–175, 2005.

[139] J. Peccoud and B. Ycart. Markovian modelling of gene product synthesis. *Theor. Pop. Biol.*, 48:222–234, 1995.

[140] K. Polach and J. Widom. A model for the cooperative binding of eukaryotic regulatory proteins to nucleosomal target sites. *J. Mol. Biol.*, 258:800–812, 1996.

[141] N. Price, J. Papin, C. Schiling, and B. Palsson. Genome-scale microbial *in silico* models: the constraint-based approach. *Trends Biotechnol.*, 21:162–169, 2003.

[142] M. Ptashne. *Genetic Switch: Phage Lambda Revisited*. 3rd ed. Cold Spring Harbor Laboratory Press, New York, 2004.

[143] A. Raj, C. Peskin, D. Tranchina, D.and Vargas, and Tyagi S. Stochastic simulations of the mammalian circadian clock. *Science*, 4:853–865, 2006.

[144] C. Rao, D. Wolf, and A. Arkin. Control, exploitation and tolerance of intracellular noise. *Nature*, 420:231–237, 2002.

[145] J. Raser and E. O'Shea. Control of stochasticity in eukaryotic gene expression. *Science*, 304:1811–1814, 2004.

[146] T. Raveh-Sadka, M. Levo, and E. Segal. Incorporating nucleosomes into thermodynamic models of transcription regulation. *Genome Res.*, 19:1480–1496, 2009.

[147] E. Renshaw. *Modelling Biological Populations in Space and Time*. Cambridge Studies in Mathematical Biology, 1991.

[148] A. Renyi. Treating chemical reaction using the theory of stochastic processes. *Magya Tud. Akad. Alkalm. Mat. Int. Kzl. (Budapest)*, 2:83–101, 1953.

[149] R.C. Robinson. *Introduction to Dynamical Systems: Discrete and Continous*. American Mathematical Society, Providence, 2012.

[150] N. Rosenfeld, J. Young, U. Alon, P. Swain, and M. Elowitz. Gene regulation at the single-cell level. *Science*, 307:1962–1965, 2005.

[151] H. Saito. Regulation of cross-talk in yeast MAPK signalling pathways. *Curr. Opinion in Microbiology*, 13:677–683, 2010.

[152] M. Savageau. Comparison of classical and autogenous systems of regulation in inducible operons. *Nature*, 252:546–549, 1974.

[153] B. Schoeberl, C. Eichler-Jonsson, E. Gilles, and G. Muller. Computational modelling of the dynamics of the MAP kinase cascade activated by surface and internalized receptors. *Nat. Biotechnol.*, 20:370–375, 2002.

[154] S. Schuster, D. Fell, and T. Dankekar. A general definition of metabolic pathways useful for systematic organization and analysis of complex metabolic networks. . *Nat. Biotechnology*, 18:326–332, 2000.

[155] E. Segal, T. Raveh-Sadka, M. Schroeder, U. Unnerstall, and U. Gaul. Predicting expression patterns from regulatory sequence in *Drosophila* segmentation. *Nature*, 451:535–540, 2008.

[156] D. Senear and G. Ackers. Proton-linked contributions to site-specific snteractions of λ *cI* repressor and O_R. *Biochem.*, 29:6568–6577, 1990.

[157] E. Seneta. *Non-Negative Matrices and Markov Chains*. Springer, 1981.

[158] R. Serfozo. *Introduction to Stochastic Networks*. Springer, New York, 1999.

[159] M. Simpson, C. Cox, and G. Sayler. Frequency domain analysis of noise in autoregulated gene circuits. *PNAS*, 100:4551–4556, 2003.

[160] H. Smith. Global dynamics of the smallest chemical reaction system with Hopf bifurcation. *J. Math. Chem.*, 50:989–995, 2012.

[161] C. Soulé. Graphic requirements for multisationarity. *ComPlexUs*, 1:123–133, 2003.

[162] J. Stelling and B. Kholodenko. Signaling cascades as cellular devices for spatial computations. *J. Math. Biol.*, 58:35–55, 2009.

[163] R. Steuer, J. Kurths, O. Fiehn, and W. Weckwerth. Observing and interpreting correlation in metabolomic networks. *Bioinformatics*, 19:1019–1026, 2003.

[164] G. Stormo and G. Hartzell. Identifying protein-binding sites from unaligned DNA fragments. *PNAS*, 86:1183–1187, 1989.

[165] O. Sturm, R. Orton, M. Birtwistle, V. Vyshermisky, D. Gilbert, M. Calder, A. Pitt, B. Kholodenko, and W. Kolch. The Mammalian MAPK/ERK Pathway Exhibits Properties of a Negative Feedback Amplifier. *Science Signaling*, 3:1–7, 2010.

[166] P. Suthers, M. Dasika, V. Kumar, G. Denisov, J. Glass, and C. Maranas. A Genome-scale metabolic reconstruction of *Mycoplasma genitalium*, *i*PS189. *Plos Comput. Biol.*, 5:e1000285, 2009.

[167] P. Swain, M. Elowitz, and E. Siggia. Intrinsic and extrinsic contributions to stochasticity in gene expression. *PNAS*, 99:12795–12800, 2002.

[168] H. Taylor and S. Karlin. *An Introduction to Stochastic Modeling, Third Edition.* Academic Press, San Diego, 1998.

[169] M. Thattai and A. van Oudenaarden. Intrinsic noise in gene regulatory networks. *PNAS*, 98:8614–8619, 2001.

[170] R. Thomas. On the relation between the logical structure of systems and their ability to generate multiple steady states or sustained oscillations. *Springer Ser. Synergentics*, 9:180–193, 1981.

[171] R. Thomas and M. Kaufman. Multistationarity, the basis of cell differentiation and memory. I. Structural conditions of multistationarity and other nontrivial behaviors. *Chaos*, 11:170–179, 2001.

[172] M. Thomson and J. Gunawardena. Unlimited multistability in multisite phosphorylation systems. *Nature*, 460:274–277, 2009.

[173] R. Tomioka, H. Kimura, T. Kobayashi, and K. Aihara. Multivariate analysis of noise in genetic regulatory networks. *J. Theor. Biol.*, 229:501–521, 2004.

[174] W Tucker. The Lorenz attractor exists. *C.R. Acad. Sci. Paris*, 328:1197–1202, 1999.

[175] W. Tutte. The dissection of equilateral triangles into equilateral triangles. *Proc. Camb. Philos. Soc.*, 44:463–482, 1948.

[176] J. Tyson. *Biochemical Oscillations.* Interdisciplanary Applied Mathematics. Springer, Berlin, 2002.

[177] J. Tyson, K. Chen, and B. Novak. Sniffers, buzzers, toggles and blinkers: dynamics of regulatory and signalling pathways in the cell. *Curr. Opinion Cell Biol.*, 15:221–231, 2003.

[178] N. van Kampen. A power series expansion of the master equation. *Can. J. Phys.*, 39:551–567, 1961.

[179] N. van Kampen. The expansion of the master equation. *Adv. Chem. Phys.*, 34:245–309, 1976.

[180] N. van Kampen. *Stochastic Processes in Physics and Chemistry.* Elsevier, 2007.

[181] J. Villar and S. Leibler. DNA looping and physical constraints on transcription regulation. *J. Mol. Biol.*, 331:981–989, 2003.

[182] C. Waddington. *The Strategy of the Genes.* London: Allen and Unwin, 1957.

[183] A. Wagner and D. Fell. The small world inside large metabolic networks. *Proc. Roy. Soc. London B.*, 268:1803–1810, 2001.

[184] J. Wang, K. Ellwood, A. Lehman, M. Carey, and Z. She. A mathematical model for synergistic eukaryotic gene activation. *J. Mol. Bio.*, 286:315–325, 1999.

[185] L. Wang, Q. Nie, and G. Enciso. Non-Essential Sites Improve Phosphorylation Switch. *Bioph. Lett.*, 99:41–43, 2010.

[186] L. Wang and E. Sontag. On the number of steady states in a multiple futile cycle. *J. Math. Biol.*, 57:29–52, 2008.

[187] P. Whittle. *Systems in Stochastic Equilibrium.* Springer, New York, 1986.

[188] T. Wilhelm and R. Heinrich. Smallest chemical reaction networks with Hopf bifurcation. *J. Math. Chem.*, 17:1–14, 1995.

[189] T. Wilhelm and R. Heinrich. Mathematical analysis of the smallest chemical reaction system with Hopf bifurcation. *J. Math. Chem.*, 19:111–130, 1998.

[190] D.J. Wilkinson. *Stochastic Modelling for Systems Biology.* Chapman & Hall/CRC, Boca Raton, 2006.

[191] W. Xiong and J. Ferrell. A positive-feedback-based bistable memory module that governs a cell fate decision. *Nature*, 426:460–464, 2003.

[192] Q. Zhang and G. Yin. Structural properties of Markov chains with weak and strong interactions. *Stoch. Proc. Appl.*, 70:181–197, 1997.

Index

E. coli, 102

abundance, 53
activation energy, 112
activator, 78
affinity function, 89
affinity plot, 89
aggregated process, 47
alpha limit set, 154
Arrehnius law, 112, 117
asymptotic pseudotrajectory, 239
asymptotically autonomous , 239
asymptotically stable, 58, 165, 197, 237
attractor, 163, 172
    Lorenz, 161
    strange, 161
auto-correlation function, 202
auto-regulation, 100

basin of attraction, 164
Bendixson, 159
Bernoulli r.v., 16, 83, 84, 90, 113, 134
binding capacity, 82
binding curve, 81, 87, 89
binding free energy, 111
binding polynomial, 80
binding rate, 5
binomial random variable, 16
birth and death processes, 8
Boltzmann machine, 85, 99, 107, 117

Cauchy-Lipschitz, 142
    Theorem, 143
chaos, 159

Chapman-Kolmogorov equation, 27
charge capacity, 140
chemical complex, 206
cI gene, 102
coefficient of variation, 25
complex balanced reaction network, 209
confluent hypergeometric function, 41, 222
cooperative, 113
cooperativity index, 93, 133, 134
covariance matrix, 195, 196
cro gene, 102
cycle
    limit, 155

deficiency, 208
density dependent process, 186
detailed balance, 37, 44, 109, 112
deterministic mass action system, 208
differential equation
    nonautonomous, 145
    of order p, 145
differential equations, 139
    linear, 169
dimerisation, 46, 221
divergence, 150
dose response curve, 92
dynamical systems, 139

entropy, 43, 134
enzyme kinetics, 40, 49, 65, 213
epigenetic landscape model, 191
equilibrium, 62, 153, 192

equilibrium constant, 18, 110
eukaryotic regulation, 111
exchangeable random variables, 84
exponential distribution, 10
Eyring model, 117

fast time-scale, 46
ferromagnetic, 85
first-order reaction network, 54, 212
Fisher information, 216
FKG inequality, 87
flow, 146, 238
fluctuation dissipation theorem, 197
free energy, 83, 111

Gaussian process, 194
general transcription factor, 77
generating function, 57
generator matrix, 33
genetic switch, 101, 102
geometric random variable, 16
GHS inequality, 89
Gibbs measure, 43, 83
Gillespie direct method, 38
gradient vector field, 163
Gronwall lemma, 144

harmonic oscillator, 148
Hartman-Grobman
    theorem, 181
Hastings, 44
heteroclinic
    cycle, 181
heteroclinic cycle, 155
Hill coefficient, 90
Hill exponent, 78
Hill function, 78
Hill plot, 90
histone, 120
holoenzyme, 113
Hopf bifurcation, 215
Hyperbolic
    matrice, decomposition, 171

i.i.d., 31
incidence matrix, 211
indirect cooperativity, 119
initiation, 77
input functions, 78
interaction graph, 192
invariant measure, 33
invariant probability measure, 34
invariant set, 154
irreducible, 33
Ising model, 85

Jacobian matrix, 150, 193

Kolmogorov equation, 11, 28, 30
Koshland cooperativity measure, 93

lac operon, 102
large deviations theory, 134
Lasalle principle, 163
law of mass action, 186
ligand, 79
linear differential equations
    in dimension two, 173
linear noise approximation, 185
linkage class, 206
Liouville formula, 150
logistic equation, 139
Lorenz, 160
Lotka-Volterra, 140, 161, 165, 166
Lyapunov
    function, 166
Lyapunov equation, 58, 59, 194, 197,
    237, 238
Lyapunov function, 162
lysogenic mode, 102
lytic mode, 102

Malthus, 139
manifold
    stable, 176
        theorem, 178
    unstable, 176

MAPK, 73
mass action kinetics, 34, 60
mass action principle, 7, 112, 205
mass transport, 67
master equation, 11, 12, 30, 221
matrix exponential, 169
matrix tree Theorem, 117
matrix tree theorem, 35, 210
May and Leonard system, 156, 181
Metropolis chain, 43, 110
Michaelis Menten, 66, 205, 216
Monod-Wyman-Changeux model, 122
multinomial, 60
multistationarity, 215
multivariate normal, 195

negative feedback loop, 5, 61, 100, 102
network topology, 58
neural network, 85
noise frequency range, 203
nucleation, 113

omega limit set, 154

partial differential equation, 57
particle system, 66
partition function, 43, 83
pathway, 113
periodic orbit point, 153
Perron-Frobeniues theorem, 35
persistence, 168
phage lambda, 85, 102, 117, 192
phase portrait, 146, 148
phenotype, 102, 191
phosphatase, 69
phosphorylation, 69
Poincaré-Bendixson theorem, 159
Poisson, 16
Poisson distribution, 13, 60
Poisson process, 31
positive feedback loop, 5, 100
predators-prey, 140
principal component, 198

prokaryote, 102
propensity function, 54, 187, 192, 207
protein burst, 199
protein kinase, 69
protein network, 69
protein phosphatase, 69

quasi-equilibrium, 46

reaction channels, 54
reaction-diffusion, 74
reference system, 84
repressor, 78
reversible, 37
ribosome, 199
RNA polymerase II, 113

saddle, 172
semiflow, 238
signalling network, 69
signalling time, 71
simulation, 38
sink, 172
source, 172
spanning tree, 35
spectral radius, 36
stable equilibrium, 165
stable matrix, 197, 237
steady state, 15, 18, 21, 34, 40, 226
steepness, 93
stepwise binding constants, 95, 96
stochastic matrix, 36
stoichiometric matrix, 54, 187, 200, 211
stoichiometric subspace, 208
strange attractor, 159
substrate, 40, 49
synergy, 110

Thomas conjecture, 192
thresholding, 131
time-continuous Markov chain, 27
trait, 191

transactivator, 110
transcription, 77
transcription factor, 6, 22, 77, 110
transcription network, 77
transcription rate, 99, 115
transduction, 69
transition probability, 27
tryptophan, 65

ultrasensitivity, 131
unstable equilibrium, 165

variational equation, 150
vector field, 188
vector fields, 139
Verhulst, 139
Volterra principle, 140

weakly reversible, 206

Zebra, 110
zero-range process, 67

Printed and bound by CPI Group (UK) Ltd, Croydon, CR0 4YY

23/10/2024

01777673-0006